D1481831

OLDER ADULTS WITH HIV:
AN IN-DEPTH EXAMINATION
OF AN EMERGING POPULATION

HIV/AIDS – MEDICAL, SOCIAL AND PSYCHOLOGICAL ASPECTS SERIES

Older Adults with HIV: An In-Depth Examination of an Emerging Population
Mark Brennan, Stephen E. Karpiak, R. Andrew Shippy and Marjorie H. Cantor (Editors)
2009. ISBN: 978-1-60876-054-1

HIV/AIDS – MEDICAL, SOCIAL AND PSYCHOLOGICAL ASPECTS SERIES

OLDER ADULTS WITH HIV: AN IN-DEPTH EXAMINATION OF AN EMERGING POPULATION

MARK BRENNAN
STEPHEN E. KARPIAK
R. ANDREW SHIPPY
AND
MARJORIE H. CANTOR
EDITORS

Nova Science Publishers, Inc.
New York

For permission to use material from this book please contact us:
Telephone 631-231-7269; Fax 631-231-8175
Web Site: http://www.novapublishers.com

NOTICE TO THE READER

The Publisher has taken reasonable care in the preparation of this book, but makes no expressed or implied warranty of any kind and assumes no responsibility for any errors or omissions. No liability is assumed for incidental or consequential damages in connection with or arising out of information contained in this book. The Publisher shall not be liable for any special, consequential, or exemplary damages resulting, in whole or in part, from the readers' use of, or reliance upon, this material. Any parts of this book based on government reports are so indicated and copyright is claimed for those parts to the extent applicable to compilations of such works.

Independent verification should be sought for any data, advice or recommendations contained in this book. In addition, no responsibility is assumed by the publisher for any injury and/or damage to persons or property arising from any methods, products, instructions, ideas or otherwise contained in this publication.

This publication is designed to provide accurate and authoritative information with regard to the subject matter covered herein. It is sold with the clear understanding that the Publisher is not engaged in rendering legal or any other professional services. If legal or any other expert assistance is required, the services of a competent person should be sought. FROM A DECLARATION OF PARTICIPANTS JOINTLY ADOPTED BY A COMMITTEE OF THE AMERICAN BAR ASSOCIATION AND A COMMITTEE OF PUBLISHERS.

LIBRARY OF CONGRESS CATALOGING-IN-PUBLICATION DATA

Brennan, Mark (Mark G.)
  Older adults with HIV : an in-depth examination of an emerging population / Mark Brennan ... [et al.].   p. ; cm.
  Includes bibliographical references and index.
  ISBN 978-1-60876-054-1 (hardcover : alk. paper)
  1. AIDS (Disease) in old age--United States. I. Title.
  [DNLM: 1. HIV Infections--psychology. 2. Aged--psychology. 3. Health Surveys. 4. Middle Aged--psychology. 5. Quality of Life. 6. Social Support. WC 503.7 B838o 2009]
  RA643.83.B74 2009
  362.196'9792--dc22   2009028853

Published by Nova Science Publishers, Inc. ✢ *New York*

8/22/11

CONTENTS

PREFACE

The first decade of the HIV/AIDS epidemic was defined by young gay men dying and activism. The second decade saw people of color and women account for the majority of those with HIV, as well as the development of effective drugs and the hope that HIV could become treatable or even curable. In this third decade, HIV has evolved into a chronic manageable disease. Few would have ever thought that there would be large numbers of older adults living with HIV in our lifetimes.Developing a strategy to best sustain the health and quality of life for the aging population living with HIV requires a rigorous assessment of this group's characteristics and needs. Research on Older Adults with HIV (ROAH), conducted by the AIDS Community Research Initiative of America (ACRIA), is the first step to begin to establish a valid comprehensive knowledge-base of the unique characteristics and needs of this growing population.

Chapter 1 - The first decade of the HIV/AIDS epidemic was defined by young gay men dying and activism. The second decade saw people of color and women account for the majority of those with HIV, as well as the development of effective drugs and the hope that HIV could become treatable or even curable. In this third decade, HIV has evolved into a chronic manageable disease. Few would have ever thought that there would be large numbers of older adults living with HIV in our lifetimes. Nearly fifteen years have passed since the introduction of highly active antiretroviral therapy (HAART). The effectiveness of HAART is illustrated by the extraordinary decrease in mortality rates and increased life expectancy among people with HIV. The result is an HIV-positive population that is both growing and greying. This pattern is seen throughout the U.S., yet few have internalized this evolution and the new set of challenges that it will bring forth. HIV has long been associated with youth and this mindset needs to change.

Chapter 2 - Health status of the HIV population is often defined by indicators used to measure the delivery of medical care (e.g., office visits, lab tests, treatment received, ambulatory versus hospital care, etc.). Such analyses rarely include age as a key variable. In an effort to provide some insight into the complex health status of these older adults, ROAH undertook a more comprehensive view of this population's health. These results are based on the self-report of ROAH participants.

The older adults in ROAH have been living with HIV for an average of 12.6 years, ranging from 3 months to 26 years. Half have an AIDS diagnosis[1] (51%) and of these 17% reported CD4 T cell levels below 200. Thus, the enormous success of highly-active antiretroviral treatment (HAART) is evident in these data.

Chapter 3 - The emergence of a growing older adult population living with HIV is testimony to the effectiveness of HAART, which has allowed them to live longer lives and escape what was an almost inevitable death sentence from AIDS. However, HAART is not a cure for HIV/AIDS. As these adults continue to age they will likely encounter the other illnesses associated with aging. Considerable physical health challenges remain ahead for this population. Unfortunately, many of those living with HIV also have a history of mental illness, particularly depression and anxiety. Some estimate that almost half of adults with HIV will confront mood, anxiety, and substance use disorders in their lifetime. Studies of younger persons with HIV have found rates of depressive disorders to be double that found in similar populations.

Clinical depression is defined as sadness, loss of interest or pleasure, feelings of guilt/low self-esteem, accompanied by changes in sleep, appetite, energy or concentration. It is one of the most common, yet highly untreated, mental health complaints affecting approximately 25% of adults at some point in their life. Among older adults, 1% to 4% may be diagnosed with major depression, and significant depressive symptoms may affect as many as 10%.

Chapter 4 - Following depression, abuse of or dependence on alcohol and other substances affecting mood or behavior remain one of the principal challenges for people living with HIV. The reported rates of substance use approach 50% in this population. Often substance use appears to be "self-medication" for existing, undiagnosed, or untreated mental health disorders. In turn, substance use can exacerbate these mental health issues. ROAH is one of the first studies to provide a careful inquiry into patterns of substance use among HIV-positive older adults. Studying this behavior in older adults with HIV is crucial. Research consistently shows that substance and alcohol use among persons living with HIV is associated with other mental health issues like depression, as well as poor adherence to antiretroviral therapy and greater risk for HIV infection.

Chapter 5 - The sexual lives of older adults are often minimized, ignored, or even ridiculed. In the media, sexual activity between two older adults is portrayed as infrequent and undesirable. When a comprehensive study of sexual behavior among older adults was published in the *New England Journal of Medicine* in 2007, the high rates of sexual activity were front page news in the *New York Times* and other national newspapers. To accompany their story, MSNBC ran a picture of two older people kissing, and received complaints that the picture was "disgusting" and "nauseating."

In the face of such negative stereotypes and ageist messages about their sexuality, older adults may experience conflict about their sexual desire and expression. On the one hand, older adults may feel embarrassed about a continued interest in sex, and may be left without resources to provide them with information and support about reducing the risks associated with their sexual expression. On the other hand, older adults may be motivated to maintain sexual activity as an expression of youthfulness because a diminished interest in sex may be experienced as an unwelcome indicator of "old age." Older adults may also want to remain

---

[1] A diagnosis of AIDS is given for CD4 T cell counts of less than 200.

sexually active out of a desire to sustain intimacy in both long-term and newly developing relationships.

Chapter 6 - Although HIV is treatable and manageable, the disease is chronic and incurable. HIV remains an infection surrounded by fear and myths. HIV stigma finds its roots in the images of the disease (full blown AIDS), coupled with the taboo behaviors of homosexuality and illicit sex, as well as substance use related to HIV infection. Many fear the mere presence of the illness. Others remain unaware or poorly informed about the modes of transmission and risk factors for HIV. Some believe an HIV-positive person's lifestyle led to the infection, and is the result of a moral failure, or is a punishment for sin. These myths contribute to the continued negative social attitudes, or stigma, experienced by people living with HIV and significantly inhibits those infected from disclosing their serostatus (i.e., HIV status). HIV stigma is well documented and appears to have increased. One-third of US adults report negative feelings toward HIV-positive persons, including the notion that people with HIV deserved their illness. HIV stigma fuels the risk of spreading the virus to others by creating a barrier to HIV testing because the mere thought of receiving a positive test result is psychologically overwhelming.

Chapter 7 - Significant resources have been used to understand HIV/AIDS and its effects on individuals, groups, societies and healthcare systems. Few studies have examined the informal social networks of this population which are a critical source of support as a person ages. Even less is known about how these social networks differ as a function of gender, sexual orientation, and race/ethnicity. Research shows that social networks are crucial to both physical and mental well-being for people of all ages, but especially as one grows older and encounters the challenges of managing multiple illnesses, many of which are chronic. If the informal caregiving provided by family, friends, and neighbors were replaced by formal caregivers (i.e., paid), the cost would exceed $300 billion annually. Will the aging HIV population be able to access informal caregiving and support within their social networks?

Chapter 8 - While older adults with HIV find themselves living longer lives due to the success of treatment with effective anti-retrovirals, this has not always been accompanied by parallel improvements in their quality of life. For the older adult, social support networks are critical. Yet these support networks are deficient and fragile. Many of these older adults lack the core social supports of spouse/partner and children, and have infrequent contact with other family members in the network. The assistance that some receive is largely in the form of emotional support from family and friends, but they perceive that support as being inadequate. Most older adults in ROAH live in communities of color, where cultural norms reinforce the importance of high levels of family interaction and reliance, yet such values do not translate into community support for older adults with HIV. What are the psychological consequences of this situation and how does it affect the well-being of this population?

Social isolation resulting from low levels of interaction and engagement with the social network often results in feelings of loneliness. Sometimes loneliness is experienced as a lack of intimacy or commitment to family or friends, or lack of contact or communication with others. Thus, many older adults are increasingly at risk for loneliness as they lose spouses, partners and friends, or become socially isolated due to changing life circumstances such as deteriorating health and fraility.

Chapter 9 - The majority of ROAH participants evidenced signs of depressive symptoms. However, this does not necessarily indicate they are without those psychological resources that enable them to adapt to their illness and life challenges as they age. Given the magnitude of depression among persons with HIV, it is not surprising that most research on psychological functioning has focused on such negative indicators, although some have included both positive and negative assessments. As a result, findings on positive psychological functioning in this population are limited. Because HAART has resulted in HIV becoming a chronic, manageable illness, a balance is needed to assess positive psychological functioning in this population so that we can better understand the full spectrum of their personal resources, and more optimally support adaptation and adjustment as people age with HIV.

Chapter 10 - Religion and spirituality can be critical personal resources for older adults as they adapt to a chronic illness and the challenges of aging. Religion and spirituality are overlapping concepts, but with distinct differences. Religiousness is an engagement with a belief system associated with a particular faith or creed. Definitions of spirituality include feelings of existential well-being involving transcendence over one's circumstances, feeling purpose and meaning in life, a sense of inner-integration, and connectedness with others. Further, religious and faith-based institutions are an important source of support and comfort. They are often pivotal cultural elements in the community-life of many racial and ethnic groups, particularly Latinos and African Americans.

Religion and spirituality can be a vital personal resource for people living with HIV. In one study 65% considered religion and 85% considered spirituality to have some level of importance in their lives. While research has examined the function of religion and spirituality among persons living with HIV, there are few studies that specifically assess older adults with HIV and spirituality. People living with HIV, including older adults, experience a strong need for meaning and hope. Why? Spirituality and religious beliefs and practices can assist in helping them to cope and adjust to challenges of living with this chronic yet life-threatening illness, as well as other circumstances that are viewed as unfair or without any sense of balance, such as HIV stigma, social isolation, or other problems. Siegel and Schrimshaw reported that among older persons with HIV (50 to 68 years), religious/spiritual beliefs and practices provided benefit that included emotional and spiritual support, reduced anxiety, and increased feelings of self-acceptance. Spirituality and religiousness are catalysts for people with HIV. These personal resources allow them to strengthen their connections with others and permit the activation of vitally important social support which are crucial in helping them adapt to an often arduous condition.

Chapter 11 - This chapter has documented the evolution of people living with HIV; each year there are more and more people growing older with this condition. In New York City the number of older adults over age 50 with HIV has been increasing at the rate of 2% annually. Using a conservative calculation, we have estimated that by 2015, over 50% of those living with HIV in New York City will be 50 and older. Further, the number of people living with HIV 65 and older has increased more than tenfold in the last decade. This graying of the HIV epidemic is all too often overlooked. But change is coming and it will require that policy makers, program planners, service providers, and researchers develop new paradigms to address this changing landscape.

How then can our communities provide optimal care for these older adults who have been given the hope of a long life due to the effectiveness of anti-retroviral therapies? Health care providers have focused on optimizing the medical treatment regimens needed to control HIV infection and its consequences. The effectiveness of this approach is measured in the dramatic reduction in mortality rates, the rise in CD4 immune cells and the drop in viral loads for those living with HIV. However, it is imperative that we broaden this focus to beyond the medical to address the myriad challenges faced by people growing older with HIV.

DEDICATION

GIVING A VOICE TO THOSE WHO ARE INVISIBLE...

This book is dedicated to the 1000 older adults living with HIV in New York City who completed the study instrument ROAH.
Listen to their voices.

The historic endeavor, ROAH (Research on Older Adults with HIV), was completely funded by ACRIA and through the trusting support of its Board of Directors. ROAH is the most comprehensive, large scale study of older adults living with HIV undertaken to-date. ACRIA's Executive Director, Daniel Tietz continues to provide the daily support and confidence that former Executive Director J. Daniel Stricker had initiated. ROAH is enormous and comprehensive. It represents the efforts of a large team of researchers and community members who unselfishly provided the insight and guidance needed to construct and execute a study of this depth and breadth. Their expertise, enthusiasm, and effort launched ROAH. They have continued their involvement as we analyze and disseminate ROAH's extensive data.

At its inception ROAH was guided by the experienced hand of Professor Emerita Marjorie H. Cantor. She has been a mentor, teacher, and friend who has influenced this effort profoundly. She reminds us that teachers do affect eternity. ROAH's pilot work, its formulation and execution occurred with the dedication, skill and informed insight of ROAH's Co-Principal Investigator, Robert Andrew Shippy, MA.

Most significantly, just over one year ago ACRIA was joined by a senior researcher Mark Brennan, PhD. He brings to the ROAH effort an esteemed research experience on aging issues and gerontology. He is President-elect of the State Society on Aging of New York. With his statistical skills he has made this book and other ROAH publications a reality. He epitomizes the spirit of scientific collaboration. Sharing the ROAH experience with Mark is one of the few unique and special thrills of my almost four decade research career.

We are especially grateful to Dr. Jeffrey Parsons (Chairman of Psychology Department, Hunter College of the City University of New York and his highly skilled and dedicated faculty and research staff at CHEST (Center for HIV Educational Studies and Training). CHEST is among the premier HIV prevention research groups in the U.S. Their guidance in how to gather data on substance use and sexual behavior was invaluable, strengthening the validity of ROAH's data set.

Many provided effort and support as ROAH evolved. Recruitment for ROAH was done rapidly due to the ceaseless efforts of ACRIA staff Philana Rowell. Data input, validation and cleaning was done with the essential support of a New York University honors intern, Allison Applebaum. Our intern this year, Liz Seidel, has provided watchful eyes assisting in literature and data updates, as well as assistance with proof-reading and manuscript preparation.

ACRIA's research on HIV and aging sensitized media and those infected with and affected by the disease. Since the release of the initial study findings the work of ROAH has continued to grow and evolve. This seminal community-based research has provided the basis for other ACRIA efforts which include research projects and programs that directly implement ROAH's recommendations, and most notably the launch of the ACRIA Center on HIV and Aging. These new efforts have been made possible by the generosity of private and public supporters including The Keith Haring Foundation, M•A•C AIDS Fund, The Robert Mapplethorpe Foundation, and the New York City Council. The authors of this book together with ACRIA's Board and staff are grateful for these important contributions and the life-changing work they have enabled.

Stephen E. Karpiak, PhD
Associate Director for Research
ACRIA Center on HIV and Aging

In: Older Adults with HIV
Editors: M. Brennan, S.E. Karpiak et al.

ISBN 978-1-60876-054-1
© 2009 Nova Science Publishers, Inc.

Chapter 1

THE EMERGING POPULATION OF OLDER ADULTS WITH HIV AND INTRODUCTION TO ROAH THE RESEARCH STUDY

Stephen E. Karpiak and Mark Brennan

The first decade of the HIV/AIDS epidemic was defined by young gay men dying and activism. The second decade saw people of color and women account for the majority of those with HIV, as well as the development of effective drugs and the hope that HIV could become treatable or even curable. In this third decade, HIV has evolved into a chronic manageable disease. Few would have ever thought that there would be large numbers of older adults living with HIV in our lifetimes. Nearly fifteen years have passed since the introduction of highly active antiretroviral therapy (HAART). The effectiveness of HAART is illustrated by the extraordinary decrease in mortality rates and increased life expectancy among people with HIV (see Figure 1). The result is an HIV-positive population that is both growing and greying. This pattern is seen throughout the U.S., yet few have internalized this evolution and the new set of challenges that it will bring forth. HIV has long been associated with youth and this mindset needs to change.

Between 2001 and 2007 (the latest year for which data are available), the number of people 50 years and older living with AIDS nearly doubled (see Figure 2; Center for Disease Control and Prevention [CDC] 2005; 2008). Already more than 70% of those with HIV are over age 40. Almost 27% of all people living with AIDS in the United States are over age 50. In New York City, the HIV/AIDS epicenter in the United States, 36% of the almost 110,000 people living with HIV are over age 50 and 72% are over age 40 (New York City Department of Health and Mental Hygiene, 2006). These same patterns are seen in local department of health reports across the country (Karpiak, 2008). In Illinois (2007) 32% of all people living with AIDS were over age 50. In Missouri (2006) 35% of all AIDS cases are older than age 50. In 2007, in both Wisconsin and Michigan, 38% of all those living with HIV were age 50 or older. If current trends in infection rates remain stable, in less than ten years half of all people living with HIV in the U.S. will be over age 50 (Karpiak).

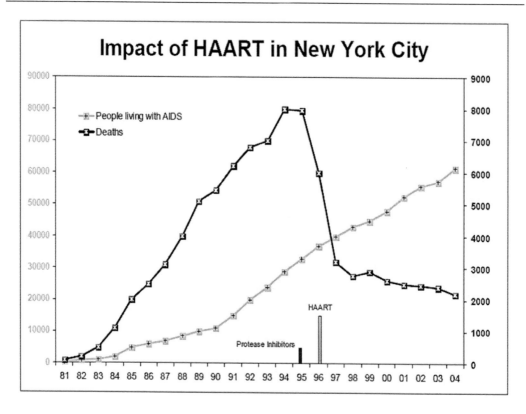

Figure 1. Changes in Mortality an Survival Rates among Persons Living with HIV in New York City following the introduction of Highly Active Antiretroviral Therapy (HAART).

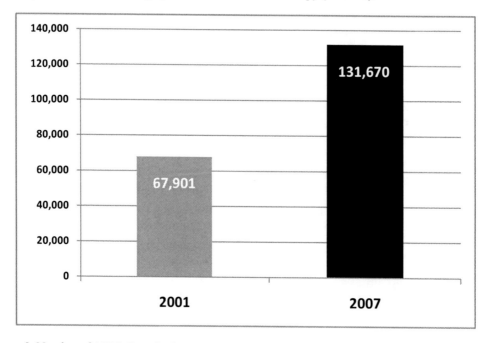

Figure 2. Number of AIDS Cases in the U.S. among People 50 Years and Older: 2001 to 2007.

Older adults with HIV are often marginalized when reporting epidemiology, conducting research and optimizing treatment programs and prevention efforts. The number of older adults with HIV may be even greater, since physicians and health officials do not perceive older adults to be at risk for HIV infection, and are not likely to test them for the virus. Consequently, under-diagnosis and late diagnosis occurs. As age increases, the likelihood of detecting the HIV infection occurring at an advanced stage increases (i.e., AIDS), making treatment and management of the disease more difficult. Because people with advanced HIV disease are highly infectious, this sets the stage for increased HIV transmission among older adults. Poor communications between health care providers and older patients do not encourage discussion about sexual behaviors and risk for HIV and other STDs because older adults are erroneously perceived as not having active sex lives (Lindau et al., 2007). Consequently, few age-appropriate HIV/AIDS risk reduction messages exist for older adults. This dearth of age-specific information causes older adults to identify themselves as being at low risk for STDs including HIV. This is a mistaken self-perception that fuels the continued spread of the virus and the stigma associated with HIV.

Many continue to see the face of AIDS being that of a gay white male, the media archetype of the 1980s. Yet in New York City, the epicenter of HIV epidemic in U.S. as well as other urban centers, the face of HIV is increasingly that of a heterosexual over the age of 50 who is a person of color, and nearly as likely to be a woman as a man. However, men who have sex with men (MSM), regardless of sexual orientation, remain the group who are the primary source of the continued transmission of HIV to both male and female partners.

ROAH THE RESEARCH STUDY

In 2002 a small not-for-profit, the AIDS Community Research Initiative of America (ACRIA), committed scarce private funds to an issue that was at best considered of little significance in the field of HIV/AIDS, namely, HIV and aging. ACRIA was uniquely positioned to conduct a high-quality, community-initiated study on a large representative sample reflecting the most current HIV epidemiology in New York City (New York City Dept. of Health and Mental Hygiene, 2006). This was possible due to ACRIA's collaborative relationships with many local AIDS service providers (ASOs) and community-based organizations (CBOs).

ACRIA's Research on Older Adults with HIV (ROAH) program is a first step in establishing a valid and comprehensive knowledge base of the unique characteristics and needs of this growing population living with HIV/AIDS. This assessment will become increasingly important in developing informed strategies to best sustain the health and quality of life for this group of older adults. ROAH has been guided by ACRIA's Associate Director for Research, Stephen Karpiak, PhD, who assembled and sustained an experienced collaborative research team. The ROAH team was joined by Marjorie Cantor, MA, Professor Emerita and Brookdale Distinguished Scholar at Fordham University, who chaired the Research Advisory Committee for the ROAH study (see Table 1). Other researchers and community members have been both advisors and collaborators with ACRIA, providing their expertise and perspectives to assist in directing the research project. In 2007 Mark Brennan,

PhD, an experienced researcher in gerontology, joined ACRIA and is engaged in the detailed analyses of the almost 1 million data points contained in ROAH.

Table 1. The ROAH Advisory Committee

ROAH Advisory Committee
Committee Chair: Marjorie H. Cantor
Professor Emerita and Brookdale Distinguished Scholar,
Graduate School of Social Service, Fordham University

Stephen Bailous Office of AIDS Policy, New York City Dept of Health	L. J. Bookhardt-Murray, MD AIDS Institute of New York State and Harlem United
David Dorfman, PhD Mt Sinai School of Medicine	Mardi Fritz NYC. Dept of Health & Mental Hygiene, Bureau of HIV/AIDS
Arlene Kochman, LCSW Yale University School of Medicine	Allen Matthews NYC Dept. of Health & Mental Hygiene, Gay & Lesbian Health
Douglas Mendez, MD Dominican Medical Association	Kathleen M. Nokes, PhD, RN, FAAN Hunter College, CUNY, Hunter-Bellevue School of Nursing
Jeffery Parsons, PhD Center for HIV/AIDS Educational Studies and Training, Hunter College	Peter Nwakeze, PhD New York Association on HIV Over 50 and Hunter College
Bobbie Sackman, MSW NYC Council of Senior Centers, Director of Public Policy	Cynthia Poindexter, PhD Fordham University Graduate School of Social Service
J. Lee Westmaas, PhD SUNY Stonybrook, Dept. of Psychology	J. Edward Shaw New York City Commission on AIDS
Nicola Di Pietro, MD, MPH Hunter College, ACRIA	Allison Applebaum, MA Boston University
Charles A. Emlet, PhD University of Washington, Tacoma	Joseph Burrage, Jr., RN, PhD University of Alabama, Birmingham
Desiree Byrd, PhD NeuroAIDS, Mt Sinai School of Medicine	Karen Fredriksen-Goldsen, PhD University of Washington, Seattle
Richard J. Havlik, MD. NIH, National Institute of Aging, Retired	

The initial release of the Research on Older Adults with HIV effort (ROAH) in 2006 caused an enormous media response followed by an increased awareness by academia, healthcare and government entities. The findings on this sample of almost 1000 New York City residents age 50 and over living with HIV show that this aging population will confront significant social, public health and medical challenges as they age.[1] ROAH is a comprehensive effort assessing basic demographics, health status, mental health, quality of life, social networks, sexual behaviors, substance use, spirituality, stigma and loneliness. The mission of ROAH is to give this group of older adults aging with HIV a needed voice and greater visibility. That voice must be heard in order to provide the care and support they will need to age successfully with decent quality of life. ROAH data should have a significant impact on the priorities for HIV/AIDS funding. A key feature of the Ryan White CARE Act, a crucial source of federal HIV/AIDS funding, has been the inclusion of community members in decision making processes which will affect their lives (New York City Department of Health and Mental Hygiene Bureau of HIV/AIDS, 2009). Older adults living with HIV should be better integrated into that process given their unique and complex needs as illustrated by ROAH. ROAH gives this aging HIV population a voice.

ROAH PARTICIPANTS AND THE SURVEY INSTRUMENT

Recruitment for ROAH did not target any specific geographic locality, neighborhood or group. Participants in ROAH were recruited from the five boroughs of New York City, by outreach coordinators utilizing ACRIA's established network of New York City-based AIDS service organizations (ASOs), public and private hospitals, and the agency's database of clients. In order to qualify for the study, participants must have been diagnosed with HIV/AIDS, age 50 or older, living in the community (i.e., not institutionalized), and sufficiently fluent in English to complete the survey instrument. From a sample of 1000 completed surveys, a final sample of 914 was obtained.[2]

The survey content was determined by the core ROAH research team (Principal Investigators Karpiak and Shippy) with guidance and input from Professor Cantor and the Research Advisory Committee. The ROAH survey instrument was constructed using existing standardized tests and encompasses six primary areas (see Appendix for details):

- Demographic Profile
- Health Status including Mental Health
- Sexual Behaviors and Substance Use
- Social Networks
- Stigma and Loneliness
- Psychological Resources including Spirituality

---

[1] Conference presentations, peer-reviewed papers, and book chapters based on the ROAH study are documented on the ACRIA website (www.acria.org), or can be obtained by contacting Drs. Brennan or Karpiak at ACRIA (mbrennan@acria.org or skarpiak@acria.org).

[2] Eighty-six surveys were discarded because they were incomplete or duplicate.

Table 2. Sociodemographic and Economic Characteristics of ROAH Participants by Gender

	Total		Men		Women		Transgender	
	M	**(SD)**	**M**	**(SD)**	**M**	**(SD)**	**M**	**(SD)**
Age[*]	55.5	(4.9)	55.7	(5.0)	55.2	(4.6)	52.0	(1.4)
	Total		Men		Women		Transgender	
	N	**%**	**N**	**%**	**N**	**%**	**N**	**%**
Age Group								
50 to 54	472	51.9	322	50.5	141	53.8	9	100.0
55 to 59	276	30.4	199	31.2	77	29.4	0	0.0
60 to 64	109	12.0	75	11.8	34	13.0	0	0.0
65 and Older	52	5.7	42	6.6	10	3.8	0	0.0
Race[***]								
Black	455	50.2	302	47.5	150	57.5	3	33.3
Hispanic	299	33.0	206	32.4	88	33.7	5	55.6
White	116	12.8	102	16.0	14	5.4	0	0.0
Asian/Pacific Islander	5	0.6	4	0.6	1	0.4	0	0.0
Native American	13	1.4	9	1.4	3	1.1	1	11.1
Multiracial	18	2.0	13	2.0	5	1.9	0	0.0
Sexual Orientation[***]								
Heterosexual	577	66.5	364	59.6	208	84.2	5	50.0
Bisexual	74	8.5	58	9.5	16	6.5	0	0.0
Homosexual	206	23.7	181	29.6	22	8.9	3	30.0
Other	11	1.3	8	1.3	1	0.4	2	20.0
Living Arrangement[***]								
Alone	631	69.7	475	75.0	151	57.6	5	50.0
Partner/Spouse	134	14.8	76	12.0	58	22.1	0	0.0
Relative	80	8.8	35	5.5	41	15.6	4	40.0
Friends	33	3.6	26	4.1	6	2.3	1	10.0
Other	27	3.0	21	3.3	6	2.3	0	0.0
Education[***]								
Some High School or Less	195	21.5	110	17.3	81	30.9	4	40.0
High School Graduate	270	29.7	186	29.2	83	31.7	1	10.0
Some College	248	27.3	179	28.1	65	24.8	4	40.0
College Graduate	195	21.5	161	25.3	33	12.6	1	10.0
Employment Status[***]								
Working	76	8.8	52	8.6	24	9.4	0	0.0
Retired	62	7.1	48	7.9	13	5.1	1	10.0
Unemployed	178	20.5	128	21.2	49	19.3	1	10.0
Homemaker	19	2.2	0	0.0	18	7.1	1	10.0
Disability	488	56.2	345	57.1	136	53.5	7	70.0
Volunteer	30	3.5	19	3.1	11	4.3	0	0.0
Other	15	1.7	12	2.0	3	1.2	0	0.0

(table continues)

Income Adequacy								
Do not have enough money	195	22.6	139	22.9	54	21.8	2	20.0
Just manage to get by	457	52.9	329	54.3	124	50.0	4	0.9
Enough with a little extra	143	16.6	89	14.7	51	20.6	3	30.0
Money is not a problem	69	8.0	49	8.1	19	7.7	1	10.0
Ever Incarcerated/Jailed (yes)**	396	45.5	297	48.9	93	36.8	6	60.0

Note. Total N = 914; Men (n = 640); Women (n = 264); Transgender (n = 10). Valid percents are reported excluding missing data.

* $p < .05$, ** $p < .01$, *** $p < .001$, One-way ANOVA for continuous variables and Chi-square tests of association for categorical variables.

ROAH was reviewed and approved by an independent review board (IRB) to ensure ethical treatment of participants. Its components, methodology and data collection details can be found in the Appendix. Data from ROAH were used to formulate the policy recommendations (See Chapter XI). Questions that ROAH raise include:

- Will an already overburdened healthcare system be able to meet the increased demands of the aging HIV/AIDS population?
- How can communities and individuals be mobilized to reduce the impending increased demands on formal care networks?
- How can limited resources be optimally utilized to address the needs of this aging population with HIV/AIDS?
- Will the aging HIV population have access to informal support from their social networks? Will their friends, families or partners provide the caregiving they will need as they age?
- How does stigma affect older adults with HIV? How can the effects of stigma be addressed for this aging population?
- Are there differences in the characteristics and needs, between genders, racial/ethnic groups, and sexual identity/orientation?
- Can those who have directed care initiatives for the HIV population embrace the known and tested paradigms which are intrinsic to achieving successful aging? Can the medical model evolve into one that is more responsive to those aging with HIV?

ROAH's large sample size provides a unique opportunity to explore how aging with HIV may differ among the major subpopulations of older HIV-positive adults. Gender, race/ethnicity, and sexual orientation[3] are the major factors examined in this book. Where statistically or clinically significant differences exist, they will be noted. While there are important distinctions among these groups that affect how policies and programs should be designed to address the needs of this population, HIV emerges as an equalizer. There is a powerful commonality in the life experience of these aging adults that minimizes factors such as sexual identity, race, culture, and gender.

---

[3] Our analysis of gender includes men, women, and transgender older adults living with HIV. While there were only 10 persons who self-identified as transgender in the ROAH sample, we felt it was important to report whatever information was available given the dearth of research that addresses the needs of this group.

DEMOGRAPHIC PROFILE: WHO ARE THEY?

The demographic profile of the ROAH respondents reflects the current epidemiological HIV data for New York City (New York City Dept. of Health & Mental Hygiene, 2006). The ROAH sample consisted of 640 men (70%), 264 women (29%), and 10 who identified as transgender (1%). The average age of ROAH participants was 55.5 years, most were between the ages of 50 to 54 (52%), and 18% were age 60 or older (see Table 2).

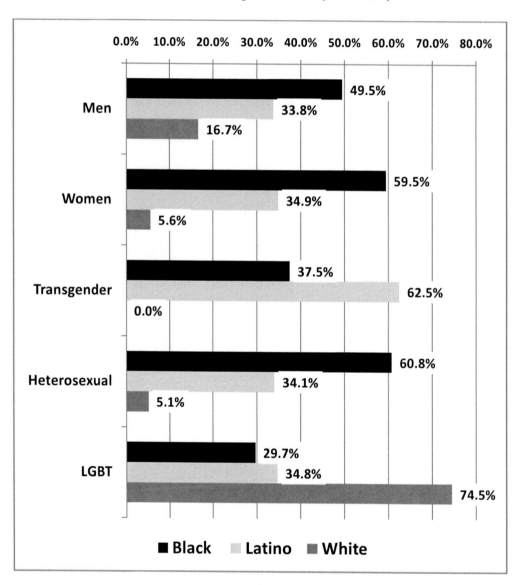

Figure 3. Gender and Sexual Orientation by Race/Ethnicity in the ROAH Sample.

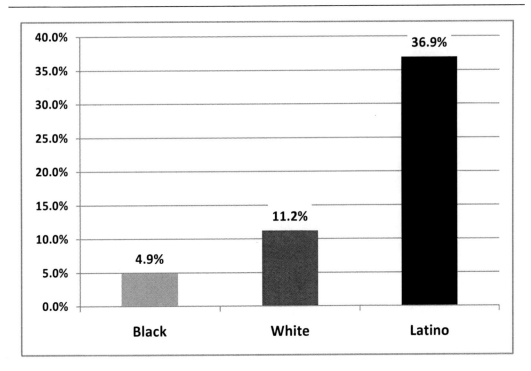

Figure 4. Proportion of Foreign-born by Race/Ethnicity.

Half of the respondents were non-Hispanic Black (hereafter referred to as Black), a third Latino, and 13% non-Hispanic White (hereafter referred to as White). The remaining 4% identified as Asian/Pacific Islander, American Indian, or multi-ethnic.[4] Regarding sexual orientation, 67% of the participants self-identified as heterosexual, 9% bisexual, and 24% homosexual. Women and heterosexuals were significantly more likely to be either Black or Latino compared to men or older LGBT adults with HIV (see Figure 3). Men made up a significantly greater proportion of the LGBT group as compared with heterosexuals (86% and 64%, respectively). The vast majority, (83%) of the participants were born in the U.S. As expected, older Latinos with HIV were significantly more likely to be foreign-born (37%) as compared with Whites (11%) or Blacks (5%; see Figure 4). In addition, older LGBT adults with HIV were significantly more likely to be foreign-born (21%) as compared with heterosexuals (15%).

A substantial proportion (71%) of the ROAH participants lived alone and 29% lived with others. Only 14% lived with a partner, 4% lived with a child, and the remaining 12% lived with a friend or other relative. As a point of comparison, only 35% of New Yorkers 65 and older live alone (New York City Department for the Aging, 2009), half the rate of those over 50 living with HIV. Men and transgender older adults were more likely to live alone (76% and 70%, respectively) than were women (58%). Additionally, LGBT persons were more likely to live alone (80%) than heterosexuals (67%). However there was no significant difference among the racial/ethnic groups. The high proportion of people who live alone, including women and heterosexuals, has significant implications regarding the need for assistance from both the informal and formal care providers as this population ages.

---

[4] Due to the small numbers in the other groups, analyses by race/ethnicity focused on differences between non-Hispanic Blacks, Hispanics/ Latinos, and non-Hispanic Whites.

When asked if they had ever been in jail 46% of the ROAH sample replied yes (49% of men and 37% of women). Heterosexuals were significantly more likely to report a history of incarceration (56%) as compared with LGBT older adults (24%). About one-half of Latinos and Blacks reported a history of incarceration (48% and 51%, respectively) as compared with 20% of Whites.

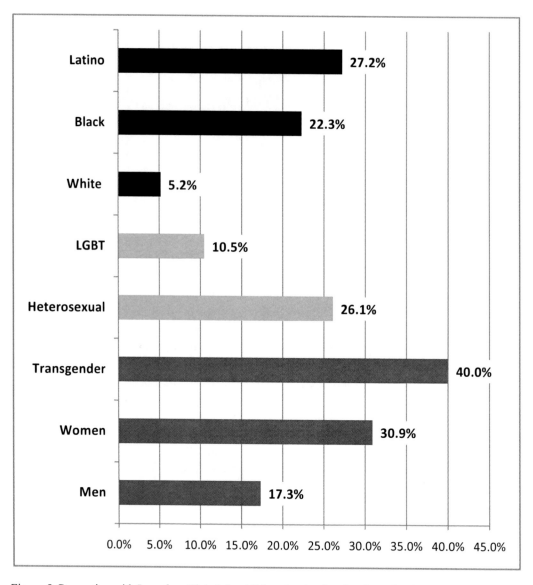

Figure 5. Proportion with Less than High School Education by Gender, Sexual Orientation, and Race/Ethnicity among Older Adults with HIV.

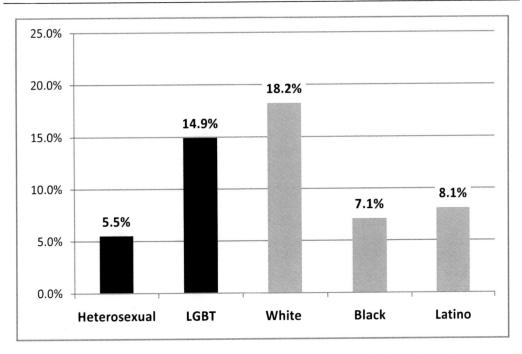

Figure 6. Proportion of ROAH Respondents Currently Working by Sexual Orientation and Race/Ethnicity.

EDUCATION, DISABILITY AND INCOME

The education level of the study group is similar to that of the general population of New York City. Three-quarters of the participants had graduated high school, and 46% had at least some college experience (see Table 2). Thirteen percent of the participants were college graduates and 9% had graduate degrees. There were significant differences in educational attainment among the major subgroups of older adults living with HIV (see Figure 5). To illustrate, transgender older adults and women were more likely than men to have not completed high school. People who identified as LGBT (i.e., primarily gay men and lesbians) were more likely to have completed high school compared to heterosexuals. Whites were also more likely to have graduated from high school compared to either Black or Latinos.

The majority of ROAH participants indicated that they were not working; 21% were unemployed, 56% were on disability, and 7% were retired. Nine percent were currently employed and 4% were volunteers (see Table 2). The proportion that was on disability did not vary among the gender, racial/ethnic and sexual orientation subgroups, but there were significant differences in the proportions working in each group correlated with participants' levels of education. Thus, men and women were more likely to be working compared with transgender adults (see Table 2). Older adults who identified as LGBT were approximately three times as likely to be working as heterosexuals. Whites were the most likely to report they were currently working (see Figure 6).

The responses to questions of income adequacy reflect the fact that most of this population is not working and 83% are Medicaid dependent. When describing their current income, 53% reported having "just enough to get by" and 23% said stated that they "do not have enough to make ends meet." Only one-quarter of the sample reported having adequate incomes (see Table 2). Reflecting differences in employment status, older adults with HIV who were LGBT were significantly more likely to respond having adequate incomes (i.e., "enough money/little extra" or "money not a problem"; 32%) as compared with their heterosexual counterparts (21%).

In summary, the profile of ROAH respondents reflects the changing face of HIV in the United States. An epidemic that got its foothold in the gay male population in the 1980s largely affects communities of color in the present day (New York City Department of Health and Mental Hygiene, 2006). Heterosexual women make up a significant proportion of current people living with HIV. Responses by ROAH participants to questions about education, income adequacy and work status find many who are at the lower end of the socioeconomic spectrum. Finally, the high proportion who lives alone suggests that many in this population may need greater socialization and social support. Without functional or viable connections to other people these older adults with HIV are vulnerable, lacking access to social resources that will be essential as they age.

REFERENCES

CDC [Center for Disease Control and Prevention]. (2005). Table 10: Estimated numbers of persons living with AIDS, by year and selected characteristics, 2001-2005 – United States and dependent areas (Revised June 2007). Retrieved March 20, 2009 from the World Wide Web: http://www.cdc.gov/hiv/topics/surveillance/resources/reports/2005 report/pdf/table10.pdf.

CDC [Center for Disease Control and Prevention]. (2008). AIDS cases by age. Retrieved March 20, 2009 from the World Wide Web: http://www.cdc.gov/hiv/topics/ surveillance/basic.htm#aidsage.

Karpiak, S. E. (October, 2008). HIV and aging: What we have learned and what we must know. Keynote address presented to the Midwest AIDS Training and Education Center Symposium, *HIV and Aging*. St. Louis, MO, October 24, 2008.

Lindau, S. T., Schumm, L. P., Laumann, E. O., Levinson, W., O'Muircheartaigh, C. A., & Waite, L. J. (2007). A study of sexuality and health among older adults in the United States. *New England Journal of Medicine, 357*, 762-74.

New York City Department for the Aging. (2009). Quick facts on the elderly in New York City. Retrieved March 20, 2009 from the World Wide Web: http://www. ci.nyc.ny.us/html/dfta/downloads/pdf/quickfacts.pdf.

New York City Department of Health and Mental Hygiene. (2006). HIV Epidemiology Program 1st Quarterly Report, Vol. 4(1). Retrieved January 31, 2006 from the World Wide Web: http://www.nyc.gov/html/doh/downloads/pdf/dires/dires-2006-report-qtr1.pdf

New York City Department of Health and Mental Hygiene Bureau of HIV/AIDS. (2009). Ryan White Care Act Reauthorization. Retrieved March 23, 2009 from the World Wide Web: http://www.nyhiv.org/pdfs/CDC-HRSA_Public_Comments_9-12-03_Final_ Version.pdf.

U.S. Bureau of the Census. (2000). Older (55+) Population Data. U.S. Washington, DC: Author.

In: Older Adults with HIV
Editors: M. Brennan, S.E. Karpiak et al.

ISBN 978-1-60876-054-1
© 2009 Nova Science Publishers, Inc.

Chapter 2

HEALTH STATUS, COMORBIDITIES, AND HEALTH-RELATED QUALITY-OF-LIFE

Richard J. Havlik

Health status of the HIV population is often defined by indicators used to measure the delivery of medical care (e.g., office visits, lab tests, treatment received, ambulatory versus hospital care, etc.). Such analyses rarely include age as a key variable. In an effort to provide some insight into the complex health status of these older adults, ROAH undertook a more comprehensive view of this population's health. These results are based on the self-report of ROAH participants.

The older adults in ROAH have been living with HIV for an average of 12.6 years, ranging from 3 months to 26 years. Half have an AIDS diagnosis[1] (51%) and of these 17% reported CD4 T cell levels below 200. Thus, the enormous success of highly-active antiretroviral treatment (HAART) is evident in these data.

HIV-RELATED HEALTH STATUS

Consistent with New York State standards of care for people living with HIV, the majority of participants (88%) visit their primary healthcare provider every 3 to 4 months, with 85% being currently on HAART. Most patients receive care in public hospitals, clinics, or AIDS service organizations (81%). There are no evident differences in access to treatment among the major racial and ethnic groups or between men and women. Almost one-third (29%) utilize some form of complementary or alternative medicine (CAM).

CD4 cell counts, a measure of HIV disease severity and immune system status, were lower on average in Whites (449) compared to Blacks (492) and lowest in Latinos (313). However, Whites were the most likely to report an AIDS diagnosis (68%) compared to Blacks (46%) and Latinos (52%). It is important to note that Whites in ROAH are largely gay men (67%) who were historically the first group affected by HIV. It is not surprising that this

---

[1] A diagnosis of AIDS is given for CD4 T cell counts of less than 200.

group had the longest history of living with HIV (M = 15 years) and explains in part the higher prevalence of AIDS diagnoses in that group. Similarly, men have a higher frequency of an AIDS diagnosis and lower CD4 levels when compared to women regardless of sexual orientation.

Heterosexual intercourse emerges as the prevailing mode of HIV transmission in the older population living with this condition at present. When asked how they were infected with HIV, 29% reported vaginal intercourse, followed by 26% who said it was from sharing needles (intravenous drug use or IDU), and lastly 23% who indicated anal sex. The remainder reported more than one source, or was unsure. Sixty-one percent of the ROAH participants who tested HIV positive in the last 5 years reported vaginal sex as a mode of transmission. For those who were infected more than 10 years ago, 32% reported vaginal sex as a mode of transmission. During the same time frame, needle sharing (IDU) and anal sex declined as modes of transmission from 41% to 24% and from 32% to 13%, respectively. These changes reflect the increase in women and self-identified heterosexual men with HIV. The lower rate of HIV infection attributed to IDU reflects implementation of needle exchange programs and targeted prevention efforts.

THE CHALLENGE: MANAGING HIV AND OTHER DISORDERS ASSOCIATED WITH AGING

In many ways the disease process in HIV/AIDS patients has characteristics of accelerated aging rather than the slower age-related changes that typically occur in the general population (Deeks & Phillips, 2009). The presence of the HIV virus in younger persons over extended periods of time may mimic the "immunosenescence" seen in older persons (Bestilny et al., 2000). This accelerated process includes reduction of the number of CD4 T cells, resulting in decreased immune competence with increased vulnerability to infectious diseases and to the side effects from certain drugs. Consequently the biological age or condition of the body of an HIV/AIDS patient may be a number of years older than his or her chronological age.

People with HIV are now living long enough to experience their condition as a chronic illness (Simone & Applebaum, 2008). As people with HIV are living longer, there will likely be one, if not several, disease processes not related to HIV that they will confront due to aging, drug toxicity, and other health comorbidities (Bhavan, Kampalath, & Overton, 2008). Absent the opportunistic infections associated with AIDS and the collapse of the immune system, the advent of HAART creates an environment where medical care focuses on health care needs that go beyond those associated with HIV. As people age, HIV will no longer exclusively define the health concerns of these older individuals.

One of the fundamental research goals to studies of HIV and aging is to understand the interactions among associated and overlapping conditions, including HIV, other comorbidities (HIV-related and non-HIV related), typical aging processes, and age-related diseases. ROAH findings highlight several important issues:

1) Are the comorbidities associated with aging and HIV infection different?

2) Are the comorbidities found in the older HIV patient related to aging alone or to the interaction of the aging process, HIV infection, and the medications (especially antiretrovirals) used by the population?

3) What are the consequences of long-term HAART?

4) How will treatment of an age-related comorbidity affect HIV treatment and the converse?

5) How do these multiple treatment regimens affect the Quality of Life of older HIV patients?

HEALTH COMORBIDITIES

Because HIV/AIDS has taken on the characteristics of a chronic disease that can be treated and managed, the patient, not the disease, must be the focus of attention as choices are made to optimize health and quality of life. The occurrences of other disease conditions or comorbidities, which exist beyond the primary effects of HIV, are characteristic of the complex health status of older people living with this condition. The person aging with HIV/AIDS will confront three types of comorbidities as they age: First, there are factors of HIV/AIDS (i.e., symptoms and complications), the adverse effects of the antiretroviral treatment, and other risks based on the person's behaviors that put them at risk for HIV. Second, older adults living with HIV can expect to experience numerous physiological changes and conditions associated with aging over time. These are aging processes that almost everyone experiences with advancing years but are not usually considered as actual diseases, such as the general decline in lung and cardiac capacity. Third, there are those chronic diseases and other conditions, distinct from HIV, which affect many older adults and require complex medical supervision. Unless these conditions are managed effectively, they can result in costly disabilities and markedly reduced quality of life or death. In fact, it is likely that these three disease processes interact, namely, any single factor can be aggravated by one or both of the other factors.

ROAH collected information on comorbidities from participants by self-report to the question: "Have you experienced any of the following health problems in the past year?" It is likely that health providers have told their HIV patients about most of these conditions, although self-diagnosis may have influenced some responses. Thorough medical screening for subclinical diseases, such as hepatitis, diabetes, or hypertension, would have identified additional cases. However, the number of comorbid health conditions in this study population is probably underestimated. Comparison of comorbidity frequencies with non-HIV patients is challenging. Still, the magnitude of the comorbidities as seen in ROAH is substantial and supports the need for comprehensive medical care for this special population presently, and long-term care in the near future. The percentage of self-reported comorbid health conditions and diseases for the ROAH sample is illustrated in Figure 1.

The number of comorbidities reported ranged from 0 to 16, with 60% reporting 3 or fewer comorbidities and 9% reporting no comorbidities. However, the average number of comorbidities in the ROAH sample (3.3) is approximately 3 times as high as that seen among community-dwelling adults 70 years and older (see Figure 2; Brennan, Horowitz, & Su, 2005).

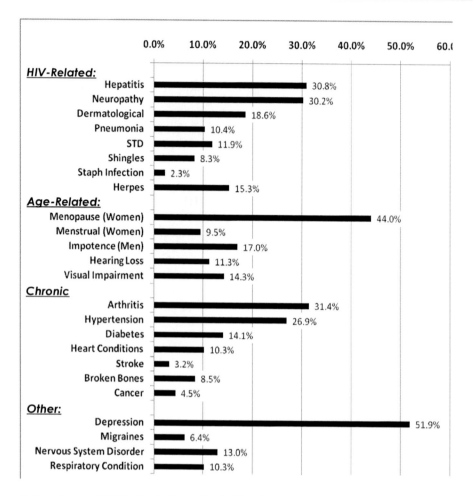

Figure 1. Prevalence of HIV-related, Age-related, Chronic, and Other Comorbidities in Older Adults with HIV.

PREVALENCE OF HIV-RELATED COMORBIDITIES IN ROAH

Hepatitis

Hepatitis was reported in 31% of the total ROAH sample, with higher percents in Blacks (34%) and Latinos (31%) when compared to Whites (19%). This distribution likely reflects the presence of concurrent hepatitis-B or hepatitis-C, possibly contracted with HIV from intravenous drug use. Liver function tests might identify even a higher prevalence of hepatitis. HIV medications can also cause liver problems, particularly Viramune (especially in women with higher CD4 counts) and Aptivus. Another possible cause of liver damage is the chronic alcohol use or over use of Tylenol (acetaminophen) for pain management. Changing HIV medications may be necessary in some cases to avoid liver damage.

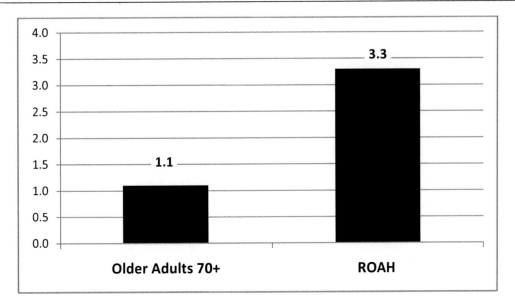

Figure 2. Comparison of Average Number of Comorbidities Reported by ROAH Respondents and Community-dwelling Older Adults.

Neuropathy

Neuropathy can result from the direct effects of the virus on the nerves in the legs and spinal cord or as a side effect from treatment with certain nucleoside reverse transcriptase inhibitor medications. The symptoms range from mild uncomfortable sensations to severe pain and loss of neurological function in the legs. In ROAH the frequency of neuropathy is highest in the White population (42%) compared to Blacks (27%) and Latinos (30%). This distribution may reflect the use of the first available antiretrovirals (ARVs) at high doses by the White gay male population. Those ARVs are now known to contribute to neuropathy. Fortunately dementia, the other nervous system complication of HIV, is a rare occurrence with current HAART, although this does not rule out the possibility of there being less obvious effects of HIV on cognitive function.

Dermatological (Skin) Problems

Skin conditions were reported by 19% of the ROAH sample, with the frequency being highest in Whites (33%). This is a non-specific category and there may be many contributing factors to these conditions. For example, specific drugs used in HAART can cause skin rashes. Abacavir (Ziagen) is associated with serious skin reaction in up to 10% of those treated, though a test is available to assess risk for this side effect. The more common conditions, such as dry skin, eczema, and seborrhea, may be associated with general aging of the skin. Treatments are aimed at alleviating symptoms and may not eliminate the condition. However treatment, especially for severe itching that may lead to skin damage and subsequent infection, is important to maintaining optimal health.

Infections

With HAART, the prevalence of opportunistic and other serious infections has been drastically reduced. Still, pneumonia, other sexually transmitted diseases (STDs), and shingles do occur. In ROAH 10% had pneumonia, 12% had an STD, and 8% reported having shingles. A vaccine to prevent shingles is now available. Staph infections were relatively uncommon at 2%. Finally, in addition to other STDs, 15% of the ROAH sample reported suffering from herpes in the previous year.

Kidney Disease

A question on kidney disease was not asked in ROAH, but recently HIV has been shown to be associated with a specific type of kidney disease known as HIV-associated nephropathy (Gupta, Eustace, Winston, et al., 2005). Although this condition is relatively uncommon, it appears to be more frequent in African Americans than in other groups. HAART has resulted in some improvement in kidney function. Viread has been linked to minor loss of function and should be avoided in people with kidney problems. Most reported problems with kidney function are complications of other conditions, such as urinary tract infections, high blood pressure, and diabetes (See below under chronic conditions).

INCREASED MANIFESTATIONS OF AGE-RELATED CONDITIONS

Body Shape

There was not a specific question about body shape on the ROAH survey; however it is an important and sensitive manifestation of accelerated aging and HIV associated lipodystrophy. With aging there is some re-distribution of fat away from the limbs and face. The protease inhibitors and other HAART drugs can result in a greater loss of fat from the face and legs and development of a "pot belly," giving an exaggerated aged appearance. The most recently developed HAART regimens, at least those being used in developed countries, have replaced earlier treatment protocols which most are more likely to have caused unwanted body changes. Unfortunately, switching to the newer drugs may not change body shape back to its prior state. Even the use of newer treatments at onset does not eliminate this problem completely, and there may be other complications. Recently, there has been increased use of products that can be injected under the skin of the face to replace lost fat cells to address facial wasting due to HIV medications. Such treatments may not be covered by medical insurance (e.g., Medicare) because they are categorized as a cosmetic procedures.

Menopause and Impotence

Menopause in women is a natural occurring process and is reported in 44 % of the female participants in ROAH. Ten percent of women reported menstrual difficulties, which may or may not be age-related. Impotence was reported by 17% of the men in ROAH. Although there are various factors affecting the ability of a man to maintain an erection, the levels of sexual potency are reduced with age in many men. In some cases this might be due to a lowering of testosterone levels or subclinical vascular disease. But in the majority of cases there is not a specific cause and could be related to psychological issues. The availability of erectile dysfunction (ED) medications has blunted such effects. The ability to overcome ED also raises the potential of not practicing appropriate HIV prevention behaviors. Adequate STI prevention information, such as the use of condoms, needs to accompany any prescription for these ED medications.

Hearing Loss and Visual Impairment

Hearing loss and visual impairment are common with aging, although there can be occupational influences which affect this type of impairment, particularly hearing loss. Hearing loss was present in 11% of the ROAH HIV population and vision loss in 14%. In the National Health Interview Survey (2000-2003) comparable figures on hearing impairment for the age group 55-64 years are higher with 22% reporting a hearing impairment, but fewer reported a visual impairment (11 %). The higher rates of visual impairment in ROAH may be due to previous exposure to opportunistic infections, as well as changes in the cardiovascular system from HIV or its treatment discussed elsewhere in this chapter (see Heart Conditions below). However, lack of comparability between the questions asked in the two surveys may also explain these differences.

CHRONIC DISEASES

Arthritis. Chronic conditions and diseases are the largest category of comorbidities mentioned by ROAH respondents. The most frequently reported disease was arthritis (31%). This figure is slightly higher than found in the National Health Interview Survey (2004) where 29% of a comparable age group (i.e., 45 to 64 years old) indicated having arthritis. It is not clear if the HIV virus itself has an effect on joints and is a cause of some forms of arthritis or its early onset.

Hypertension. Hypertension (i.e., high blood pressure) was present in 27% of the ROAH population with more Blacks (31%) reporting the disease than Whites (20 %) and Latinos, (22%). It is common to observe a rise in blood pressure at older ages due to the hardening of the arteries. This is most evident with systolic blood pressure (the top value when reported), which is associated with increased cardiovascular risk. Diastolic blood pressure (the lower number) may stabilize with age, although elevations occur and lead to a diagnosis of hypertension. Weight gain and salt intake also increase hypertension risk; consequently treatment guidelines include reductions in these two lifestyle factors. Effective treatment for hypertension with medications is available, and reduction of blood pressure has been shown to reduce the risk of heart attack and stroke. Most blood pressure drugs can be used by people taking HIV medications, although the class of drugs known as calcium channel blockers can be problematic when combined with certain protease inhibitors used in HAART.

Diabetes. Diabetes or high blood sugar (glucose) was reported in 14% of the ROAH population. This percent is comparable to adult data for ages 45-64 years from a New York City Department of Health and Mental Hygiene survey, which found that 13% reported ever being told they had diabetes. We might have expected higher rates of diabetes in ROAH due to the known side effects of HAART. Insulin is necessary for metabolizing nutrients, but is less efficient as one ages. Therefore there is a tendency for functional problems to develop in the way sugar is handled by the body. This can lead to diabetes, especially in those who are obese or have a family history of this condition. For other people, diabetes is identified only with the administration of a special glucose tolerance test, and may not be as serious a problem. If this glucose abnormality is coupled with obesity, hypertension, high triglycerides, and low HDL cholesterol (i.e., not enough good cholesterol), it is referred to as the "metabolic syndrome." Treatment with protease inhibitors has been associated with glucose intolerance. Such treatment could exacerbate a tendency toward the development of a metabolic syndrome. If possible, a switch in drug regimens may be considered. With a successful HAART regimen, however, it may be preferred to continue therapy and control glucose intolerance with weight reduction, exercise, and dietary changes. Such a strategy would also improve lipid and blood pressure abnormalities. There are also effective medications for controlling blood sugar and some can be used effectively with HAART.

Lipids (Blood Fats). The self report in ROAH did not allow for assessing the occurrence of hyperlipidemia (High blood fats), a potentially serious side effect of HAART. Researchers estimate that these metabolic side effects are common, with abnormally high cholesterol occurring in about one-fifth of patients who are on a typical HAART regimen (Friis-Moller et al., 2003). This condition causes concern since elevated cholesterol levels can predispose a person to increased risk for atherosclerosis and coronary heart disease (See Heart Conditions below).

Heart Conditions and Stroke. The presence of a heart condition was reported by 10% of ROAH respondents. Most of these reports likely reflect atherosclerosis, or hardening of the coronary arteries, which can manifest themselves as a heart attack or chest pain (angina pectoris). Another manifestation of vascular disease is stroke, which was reported at 3% in ROAH. Many earlier studies had not found a direct relationship between HIV, treatment, and coronary heart disease. However, recent reports support the conclusion that the virus alone might lead to increased risk for coronary heart disease (SMART Study Group, 2006) becoming evident as the person ages. In developed countries, the frequency of atherosclerosis and myocardial infarctions (heart attack) increases with age. This is believed to be the cumulative effect of lifestyle and genetic factors rather than simply growing older. Besides hypertension, abnormal blood lipids and diabetes, smoking is the single most powerful predictor of cardiovascular disease and cancer, especially in men (57% of ROAH participants are current smokers, while 84% report a history of smoking as compared to 24% in New York State overall). Addressing these treatable risk factors as well as providing optimal HAART therapy are the best approaches to minimizing heart attack risk.

Broken Bones. Broken bones or fractures associated with falls or other trauma are common at older ages. The ROAH population is not elderly in terms of chronological age, but one finds that 9% have suffered a fracture during the past year. The incidence of fractures in the ROAH sample is markedly higher than among comparable groups, where 1% to 3% experiences a fracture in a given year (Cauley et al., 2008). One possible explanation for ROAH's high frequency is the presence of subclinical osteoporosis or softening of the bones, which is more common with aging but is associated with other risk factors such hormonal deficiencies or dietary factors. Measurement of bone density in HIV patients suggests there is a greater loss of bone density beyond what would be expected in a non-HIV population (Bhavan, Kampalath, & Overton, 2008). It has been hypothesized that chronic inflammation associated with HIV infiltration into the tissues over many years, even at low levels, could be a contributing factor. Within limits, fractures resulting from osteoporosis can be successfully prevented with oral medications.

Cancer. Cancer frequency in ROAH was reported as 5%. Fortunately, two of the AIDS-defining cancers, Kaposi's sarcoma and non-Hodgkin's lymphoma have become less common during the period of increased HAART usage. However, invasive cervical cancer has remained a health concern for women. In addition, certain non-AIDS defining cancers have become an increasing medical problem (Crum-Chianflone et al., 2009). First among these is lung cancer, which has shown an increased occurrence in people living with HIV compared to national rates. One of the key risk factors for lung cancer is smoking, and, as indicated, smoking is common among older HIV patients; 57% in ROAH currently smoke, 84% have a history of smoking. Also, one report indicates that the duration of HIV infection may be a risk factor for lung cancer (Levine, 2008). Screening for early lung cancer in at-risk patients may be indicated as part of medical care for this aging HIV population.

Other malignant tumors of note are head and neck cancers and liver cancers. The former are associated with human papilloma virus, similar to invasive cervical cancer. This virus may be a common etiological factor for these malignancies. A vaccine program is underway in young women to prevent infections, but this strategy would not be appropriate for older HIV patients. Finally, hepatitis B and C infections are associated with an increased risk for liver tumors. A hepatitis frequency of 30% in the ROAH sample suggests increased risk and the need for medical system awareness of the potential for such malignancies in older HIV patients.

OTHER DISEASE CONDITIONS

By far, the most frequently reported comorbidity in the ROAH sample was depression, with 52% indicating problems with depression in the past year. These self-report data are in agreement with the assessment of depression included in ROAH (see Chapter III). Migraines were reported by 6% of respondents, while approximately one-in-ten suffered from unspecified nervous or respiratory conditions (13% and 10%, respectively).

SELF-RATED HEALTH

As a summary measure of overall health, ROAH participants rated their current health on a possible scale of 0-10, with higher scores indicating better health. The participants' mean score is 6.8, indicating that most consider their overall health to be at least fair or good. In many ways this measure is analogous to asking the question, "How are you feeling today?" The answer of ROAH's participants could be characterized in the range of "Not Bad" to "Good." Given the multiple challenges these individuals face in managing HIV, together with other daily life issues (i.e., stigma, isolation, loneliness, the "red-tape" of the medical system), one concludes that medical management of their HIV and programs available to them through the Ryan White Care Act have been effective to-date.

SUMMARY ON HEALTH COMORBIDITIES INFORMATION

The availability of ROAH data on self-reported comorbidities provides important documentation on the frequent occurrence of health conditions in this population. These data support the conclusion that policy makers and health care planners must acknowledge the reality that the HIV/AIDS populations is growing older and will encounter significant health care needs beyond HIV disease. This challenge must be addressed now so the medical care system will be prepared to meet this challenge in the coming decades.

HIV-RELATED QUALITY OF LIFE

For the older person living with HIV/AIDS, who is experiencing a longer life span due to HAART therapy, the quality of that extended life becomes paramount. The ROAH survey addressed this fundamental question by exploring quality of life (QoL) in five areas (Cognitive Function, Physical Function, Social function, Pain, and Energy/Fatigue) using the MOS-HIV measure (Wu et al., 1991, see Appendix). Because different numbers of items were included in each of these five assessments, scores were standardized to a range of 0 to 100 for comparison purposes with higher scores suggesting better quality of life. As seen in Figure 3, the ROAH respondents were most challenged in QoL in terms of energy/fatigue followed by pain and physical functioning respectively. In contrast, levels of cognitive and social functioning QoL were the highest among ROAH respondents. All of these scale differences were statistically significant, except for the differences between pain and physical functioning, and cognitive and social functioning.[2] Thus, the physical impact of HIV, in terms of energy and fatigue, pain and physical functioning, represent the greatest challenges to QoL among this sample of older adults with HIV.

---

[2] Standardized QoL scores were examined with paired-sample t-tests, using a Bonferonni correction for multiple comparisons in order to maintain a statistical significance level of $p < .05$.

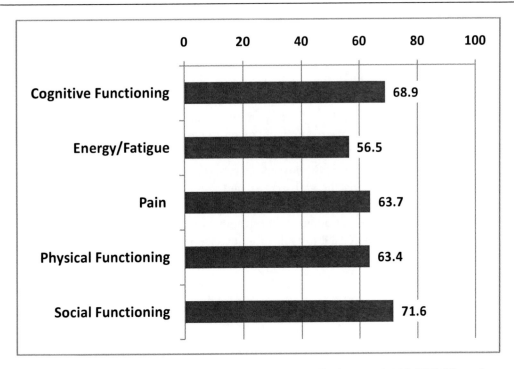

Figure 3. Comparison of Health-realted Quality of Life Standardized Scores (MOS-HIV; Wu et al., 1991) among ROAH Participants in Five Domains. All domain differences were statistically significant with the exception of cognitive function vs. social function, and pain vs. physical function.

Table 1. Correlations of Age and Health Indicators with HIV Health-related Quality of Life (QoL)

		1	2	3	4	5	6	7	8	9	10
1	Age	1.00									
2	Months Since HIV Diagnosis	.08*	1.00								
3	CD4 Count	-.02	-.15**	1.00							
4	Number Comorbidities	-.08*	.12**	.00	1.00						
5	Self-rated Health	.02	-.07*	.10**	-.33***	1.00					
6	QoL Cognitive	.10**	.04	.03	-.18***	.18***	1.00				
7	QoL Physical	-.04	-.06	.02	-.24***	.29***	.31***	1.00			
8	QoL Social	.03	-.06	-.03	-.19***	.23***	.34***	.36***	1.00		
9	QoL Pain	.11**	-.11**	.04	-.36***	.35***	.19***	.40***	.31***	1.00	
10	QoL Energy/Fatigue	.04	-.11**	.09*	-.34***	.42***	.38***	.43***	.34***	.51***	1.00

* $p < .05$, ** $p < .01$, *** $p < .001$.

Because QoL measures are highly interrelated, one anticipates that there would be associations or correlations among the five measures. In fact such associations did occur examining the QoL raw scores. For example, satisfaction with cognitive function was significantly related to the other four areas. However, correlations were modest in the range of .20 to .30. Higher correlations of .40 to .50 occurred between the more general domains of energy/fatigue and the areas of physical function, social function and pain (see Table 1).

When first investigating other correlates of these QoL measures, not surprisingly, the number of comorbid conditions, an indicator of overall disease burden, and self-reported health status correlated highly with QoL measures. Generally, the higher the numbers of comorbid conditions the lower the QoL scores, and the higher the self-rating of health, the higher the QoL scores. Interestingly, ROAH participant's age was not a significant factor affecting the QoL measures. In addition, the length of time ROAH respondents had been living with HIV/AIDS was related to QoL in an inverse manner, suggesting that the longer HIV/AIDS has been present, the lower the current life satisfaction/quality of life.

SUMMARY OF HIV-RELATED QoL

Gender and race are unrelated to QoL measures, suggesting that the HIV virus is having widespread effects across these subgroups. Other factors that cannot be altered such as length of infection, although important, also have to be accepted. The challenge is to continue to identify factors that can be modified in the lives of older people living with HIV/AIDS in order to provide programs and interventions to positively affect their health status. A good example is depression, which was common in the current sample and can be successfully treated in most cases (see Chapter III). Another broader area is the prevention and thereby reduction in the frequency or symptoms of other comorbid conditions, such as neuropathy, which can reduce QoL, to insure the best possible quality of life during the extended years of life caused by effective HAART therapy.

CONCLUSIONS

The health status of older adults living with HIV was illustrated by self-reports from the ROAH study. Of special interest is the occurrence of comorbidities reported by ROAH participants. Besides frequent depressive symptoms, other frequently reported diseases and conditions were arthritis, hepatitis, neuropathy, and hypertension. These comorbidities represent a mixture of the effects of the virus itself. While anti-retrovirals protect the immune system from collapse due to HIV infection, the virus is likely exerting effects on other organ systems and tissue metabolic activities. These HIV effects may be contributing to the seemingly early onset and severity of age associated illnesses. Because of the frequent occurrence of comorbidities in older HIV patients, the medical care team should be made aware of the need to screen and treat such conditions. The challenge is to accomplish these goals effectively within the realities of the current medical care system and reimbursement schemes. When management by the primary care team is not going well, a suitable referral should be arranged and facilitated. An ultimate goal of medical management is to assure a satisfying quality-of-life for the person aging with HIV, regardless of the HIV status and the number or severity of comorbidities. This requires a commitment to both implementing treatment approaches with a proven track-record of success, as well as further research into improved health care management of this aging HIV population (Effros et al., 2008).

REFERENCES

Bestilny, L. J., Gill, M. J., Mody, C. H., & Riabowol, K. T. (2000). Accelerated replicative senescence of the peripheral immune system induced by HIV infection. *AIDS, 14*, 771-780.

Bhavan, K. P., Kampalath, V. N., & Overton, E. T. (2008). The aging of the HIV epidemic. *Current HIV/AIDS Reports, 5,* 150-158.

Brennan, M., Horowitz, A., & Su, Y. (2005). Dual sensory loss and its impact on everyday competence. *The Gerontologist, 45,* 337-346.

Cauley, J. A., Wampler, N. S., Barnhart, L. et al. (2008). Incidence of fractures compared to cardiovascular disease and breast cancer: The Women's Health Initiative Observational Study. *Osteoporosis International, 19*, 1717-23.

Crum-Chianflone, N., Jullsiek, K. H., Marconi, V., et al. (2009). Trends in the incidence of cancers among HIV-infected persons and the impact of antiretroviral therapy: A 20-year cohort study. *AIDS, 23*(1), 41-50.

Deeks, S. G., & Phillips, A. N. (2009). HIV infection, antiretroviral treatment, ageing, and non-AIDS related morbidity: Review. *BMJ, 338,* a3172.

Effros, R. B., Fletcher, C. V., Gebo, K., Halter, J. B., Hazard,W. R., Horne, F., et al. (2008). Aging and infectious diseases: Workshop on HIV infection and aging: What is known and future research directions. *Clinical Infectious Diseases, 47,* 542-53.

Friis-Moller, N., Weber, R., Reiss, P., Thiebaut, R., Kirk, O., & Monforte, A., et al. (2003). Cardiovascular disease risk factors in HIV patients – association with antiretroviral therapy. Results from the DAD study. *AIDS, 17,* 1179-1193.

Gupta, S. K., Eustace, J. A., Winston, J. A. et al., (2005). Guidelines for the management of chronic kidney disease in HIV-infected patients: Recommendations of the HIV Medicine Association of the Infectious Disease Society of America. *Clinical Infectious Diseases, 40,* 1159-1585.

Levine, A.M. (2008). Non-AIDS-defining cancers in the era of HAART. In E.P. Seeskin, E. King, S. McGuire & T.O. Gross (Eds.) *HIV/AIDS Annual Update 2008.* Clinical Care Options, LLC.

Simone, M.J., & Applebaum, J. (2008). Management of HIV/AIDS in older adults. *Geriatrics, 63,* 6-12.

The Strategies for Management of Antiretroviral Therapy (SMART) Study Group (2006). CD4+ Count-guided interruption of antiretroviral treatment. *New England Journal of Medicine, 355,* 2283-2296.

Wu, A.W., Rubin, H.R., Mathews, W.C., Ware Jr, J.E., Brysk, L.T., Hardy, W. D., (1991). A health status questionnaire using 30 items from the Medical Outcomes Study. Preliminary validation in persons with early HIV infection. *Medical Care, 29,* 786-798.

In: Older Adults with HIV
Editors: M. Brennan, S.E. Karpiak et al.

ISBN 978-1-60876-054-1
© 2009 Nova Science Publishers, Inc.

Chapter 3

MENTAL HEALTH AND DEPRESSION

Allison Applebaum and Mark Brennan

The emergence of a growing older adult population living with HIV is testimony to the effectiveness of HAART, which has allowed them to live longer lives and escape what was an almost inevitable death sentence from AIDS. However, HAART is not a cure for HIV/AIDS. As these adults continue to age they will likely encounter the other illnesses associated with aging (see Chapter II). Considerable physical health challenges remain ahead for this population. Unfortunately, many of those living with HIV also have a history of mental illness, particularly depression and anxiety. Some estimate that almost half of adults with HIV will confront mood, anxiety, and substance use disorders in their lifetime (Bing et al., 2001; Ciesla & Roberts, 2001; Pence et al., 2006). Studies of younger persons with HIV have found rates of depressive disorders to be double that found in similar populations (Atkinson & Grant, 1994; Bing et al.; Ciesla & Roberts; Dew et al., 1997; Jin et al., 2006; Maj et al., 1994; Rabkin et al., 2000).

Clinical depression is defined as sadness, loss of interest or pleasure, feelings of guilt/low self-esteem, accompanied by changes in sleep, appetite, energy or concentration. It is one of the most common, yet highly untreated, mental health complaints affecting approximately 25% of adults at some point in their life (Ebmeier, Donaghey & Steele, 2006; Kessler et al., 2003; Noble, 2005). Among older adults, 1% to 4% may be diagnosed with major depression, and significant depressive symptoms may affect as many as 10% (Blazer, 2002; 2003; U. S. Department of Health and Human Services, 1999).

DEPRESSION IN ROAH

In ROAH, depression was assessed using the Center for Epidemiologic Studies Depression Scale (CES-D; Radloff, 1977), one of the most commonly used standardized tools to assess depressive symptoms in adults. The CES-D yields a symptom score that can range from 0 to 60; higher scores indicate greater depressive symptoms. In the general population, CES-D scores over 16 indicate clinically significant depressive symptoms. Scores between 22 and 24 have been used to indicate a high likelihood of a major depressive disorder

(Lewinsohn et al., 1997; Lyness, et al., 1997; Roberts, Lewinsohn, & Seeley, 1991). We used 23, the midpoint of these values, as a threshold of likely major depression in the ROAH study.

In ROAH the average CES-D score was 20.0 (*SD* = 10.7). As seen in Figure 1, almost 40% of those in ROAH met the threshold for severe depression (CES-D scores of 23 or more), while 24% had moderate levels of depressive symptoms (scores of 16 to 22). The remaining 37% had no evidence of significant depression (scores lower than 16; see Figure 1). These data indicate that aging HIV-positive adults experience remarkably high levels of depression, at a rate almost five times higher than the general New York City population (Galea et al., 2002). As shown in Figure 2, the level of depressive symptoms found in ROAH is two to three times that reported in other studies of middle-age and older adults (Gump et al., 2005), or among older adults with vision loss, another group characterized by higher than average levels of depression (Horowitz, Brennan, Reinhardt, & MacMillan, 2006).

Group Differences in Depression

In ROAH, we did not observe any significant differences in depressive symptoms between men, women and transgender older adults with HIV, or between LGBT individuals and heterosexuals. ROAH did find significant differences in depression by race/ethnicity.[1] As shown in Figure 3, Latinos had significantly higher levels of depressive symptoms (21.3) compared to Blacks (19.0).

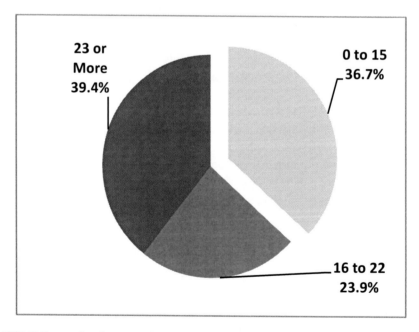

Figure 1. CES-D Depressive Symptom Score Breakdown among Older Adults with HIV. Scores of 16 to 21 indicate clinically significant depressive symptoms, while scores of 23 or higher indicate a likely diagnosis of depression.

---

[1] $F(2, 860) = 4.71, p < .01$

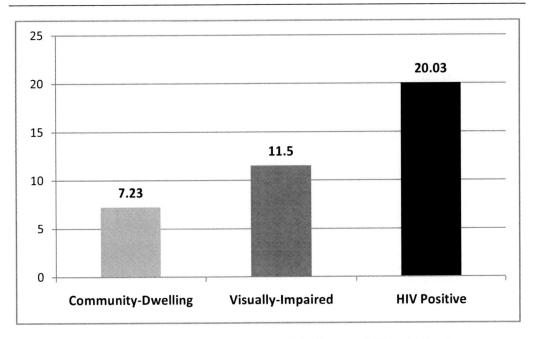

Figure 2. Comparison of Average CES-D Scores among Middle-age and Older Adults who are Community-dwelling, Visually-Impaired, or Living with HIV in ROAH. Data on Community-dwelling adults and visually impaired adults were obtained from Gump et al. (2005) and Horowitz et al. (2006), respectively.

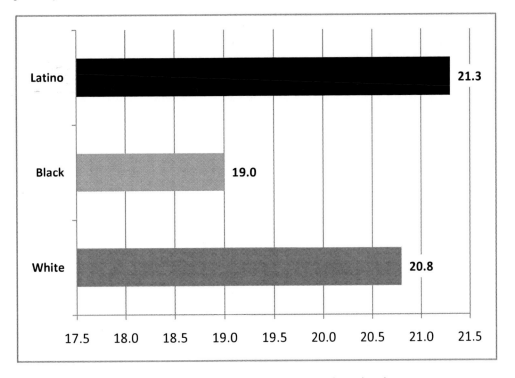

Figure 3. CES-D Depression Scores in ROAH among Whites, Blacks and Latinos.

Other research on younger HIV-positive groups has suggested that depression in this population may vary between men and women (Applebaum et al., 2009; Ickovics et al., 2001; Tostes, Chalub, & Botega, 2004; Tryznka & Erlen, 2004). Others have found elevated rates of depression in African Americans living with HIV (Johnson, Cunningham-Williams & Cottler, 2003; Lichtenstein, Laska & Clair, 2002; Lyon & Munro, 2001; Moneyham, Shacham, Basta & Reece, 2008), and in gay and bisexual men (Berg, Mimiaga, & Safren, 2004; 2008; Dickey, Dew, Becker & Kingsley, 1999). Considering that ROAH is the first large-scale study to examine depression among older adults with HIV, our current findings suggest that depression may manifest itself in other ways in this aging population, and point to the need for more in-depth research with this group as well as an assessment of present standards of care. The high rates of depression found among older Latinos with HIV likely reflects recent reports that this group has been underserved, particularly by mental health care providers (Brennan et al., 2005).

DOUBLE JEOPARDY: DEPRESSION AND HIV

Depression can directly affect the progression of a physical illness. Among older adults whose immune systems are already compromised and weakened by HIV, depression may increase that vulnerability to infectious disease by further suppressing the body's defenses. Depressive symptoms, especially in the presence of severe stress, may cause decreases in vital immune system cells, such as CD4 cells and lymphocytes (Kopnisky, Stoff, & Rausch, 2004). Similarly, elevated symptoms of depression and the presence of severe stress are associated with a faster progression to AIDS (Kopnisky, et al.; Leserman, 2003).

Depression can adversely affect many day-to-day activities, such as self-care behaviors, and most importantly adherence to HIV medications (Chesney, 2000; Holzemer et al., 1999; Mehta, Moore, & Graham, 1997; Singh et al., 1996; Tryznka & Erlen, 2004; Wagner, Kanouse, Koegel & Sullivan, 2003). Failure to adhere to HIV treatments results in poor management of this condition and the emergence of treatment-resistant strains of the virus (Tryznka & Erlen). Arguably, the impact of depression on health is a greater concern for older adults with HIV since they also need to adhere to medications to treat other serious and chronic health conditions associated with aging.

SUMMARY AND CONCLUSIONS

There is no single identifiable factor that accounts for these high levels of depressive symptoms found in the ROAH sample. The ROAH cohort is actively engaged in medical care, and arguably has access to a myriad of support and treatment options for mental health disorders. Depression *is* a manageable and treatable condition. One reason for the high levels of depression in ROAH may be the difficulty in recognizing depression when symptoms are not typical or are easily confused with HIV, other physical ailments and the aging process itself. For example, many people living with depression do not necessarily feel sad; rather, depression is often expressed by agitation and irritability. In addition, many of the physical symptoms of depression (poor appetite, lack of energy) are also symptoms associated with

HIV as well as the aging process. Many HIV physicians are focused on the medical treatment of HIV, and may view depressive symptoms as an expected and tolerable reaction to living with the virus. In many cases, this marginalizes the mental health needs of this growing group of older adults.

There is a stigma associated with mental illness similar to that surrounding HIV. Older adults continue to view depression as shameful or as a sign of weakness that should not be acknowledged. Stigma associated with mental illness may be even higher in communities of color (Brennan et al., 2005). There is often the mistaken belief that nothing can be done, and so depression can be particularly destructive for older adults who are less likely to seek treatment. Physicians often fail to ask the questions that will identify and diagnose depression in their older patients. In the era of effective HAART, it is vital that health care providers be prepared to assess and treat the myriad physical and mental health conditions that adults aging with HIV will face. The co-occurrence of HIV and depression is a formula for continued strain on the immune system. Timely identification, treatment and monitored management of depression among adults with HIV, regardless of age, are indispensable for optimal management of this condition.

REFERENCES

Applebaum, A., Richardson, M., Brady, S., Brief, D. & Keane, T. (2009). Gender and other psychosocial factors as predictors of adherence to highly active antiretroviral therapy (HAART) in adults with comorbid HIV/AIDS, psychiatric and substance-related disorders. *AIDS and Behavior, 13*, 60 – 65.

Atkinson, J. & Grant, I. (1994). Natural history of neuropsychiatric manifestations of HIV disease. *Psychiatric Clinics of North America, 17*, 17 – 33.

Berg, M., Mimiago, M. & Safren, S. (2004). Mental health concerns of HIV-infected gay and bisexual men seeking mental health services: An observational study. *AIDS Patient Care and STDs, 18*, 635 – 643.

Berg, M., Mimiaga, M. & Safren, S. (2008). Mental health concerns of gay and bisexual men seeking mental health services. *Journal of Homosexuality, 54*, 293 – 396.

Bing, E., Burnam, M., Longshore, D., Fleishman, J., Sherbourne, C., London, A. et al. (2001). Psychiatric disorders and druguse among human immunodeficiency virus-infected adults in the United States. *Archives of General Psychiatry, 58*, 721–728.

Blazer, D. G. (2002). *Depression in later life,* (3rd ed.). New York: Springer.

Blazer, D. G. (2003). Depression in late life: Review and commentary. *Journal of Gerontology: Series A: Biological Sciences and Medical Sciences: 58*, 249-265.

Brennan, M., Vega, M., Garcia, I., Abad, A., & Friedman, M. B. (2005). Meeting the mental health needs of elderly Latinos affected by depression: Implications for outreach and service provision. *Care Management Journals, 6* (2), 98-106.

Chesney, M. (2000). Factors affecting adherence to antiretroviral therapy. *Clinical Infectious Disease, 30*, S171 – S176.

Ciesla, J.A. & Roberst, J.E. (2001). Meta-analysis of the relationship between HIV infection and risk for depressive disorders. *American Journal of Psychiatry, 158*, 725 – 730.

Courteny-Quirk, C., Wolitski, R. J., Parsons, J. T., Gomez, C. A., & Seropositive Urban Men's Study Team. (2006). Is HIV/AIDS stigma dividing the gay community? Perceptions of HIV-positive men who have sex with men. *AIDS Education & Prevention, 18*(1), 56-67.

Dew, M., Becker, J., Sanchez, J., Cladararo, R., Lopez, O., Wess, J., Dorst, S. & Banks, G. (1997). Prevalence and predictors of depressive, anxiety and substance use disorders in HIV-infected and uninfected men: A longitudinal evaluation. *Psychological Medicine, 27*, 395-409.

Dickey, W., Dew, M., Becker, J. & Kingsley, L. (1999). Combined effects of HIV-infection status and psychosocial vulnerability on mental health in homosexual men. *Social Psychiatry and Psychiatric Epidemiology, 34*, 4 – 11.

Ebmeier, K., Donaghey, C. & Steele, D. (2006). Recent developments and current controversies in depression. *Lancet, 367*, 153 – 167.

Galea, S., Ahern, J., Resnick, H., Kilpatrick, D., Bucuvalas, M., Gold, J., & Vlahov, D. (2002). Psychological sequelae of the September 11 terrorist attacks in New York City. *New England Journal of Medicine, 346*(13), 982–987.

Gump, B. B., Matthews, K. A., Eberly, L. E., Chang, Y., & MRFIT Research Group. (2005). Depressive symptoms and mortality in men. *Stroke, 36*, 98-102.

Heckman, B. D. (2006). Psychosocial differences between whites and African Americans living with HIV/AIDS in rural areas of 13 U.S. states. *Journal or Rural Health, 22*(2), 131-9.

Holzemer, W., Corless, I., Nokes, K., Eller, L., Bunch, E., Kemppinen, J., et al. (1999). Predictors of self-reported adherence in persons living with HIV disease. *AIDS Patient Care and STDs, 13*, 185 – 197.

Horowitz, A., Brennan, M., & Reinhardt, J.P., & MacMillan, T. (2006). The impact of assistive device use on disability and depression among older adults with age-related vision impairments. *Journal of Gerontology: SOCIAL SCIENCES, 61B* (5), S274-S280.

Ickovics, J. R., Hamburger, M. E., Vlahov, D., Schoenbaum, E. E., Schuman, P., Boland, R. J., & Moore, J. (2001). Mortality, CD4 cell count decline, and depressive symptoms among HIV-seropositive women. *Journal of the American Medical Association, 285* (11), 1466-1474.

Jin, H., Atkinson, H., Yu, X., Heaton, R., Shi, C., Marcotte, T. et al. (2006). Preliminary communication: Depression and suicidality in HIV/AIDS in China. *Journal of Affective Disorders, 94*, 269 – 275.

Johnson, S. D., Cunningham-Williams, R. M., Cottler, L. B. (2003). A tripartite of HIV-risk for African American women: The intersection of drug use, violence, and depression. *Drug and Alcohol Dependence, 70*(2), 169-75.

Kessler, R., Berglund, P., Demler, O., Jin, R., Koretz, D., Merikangas, K. et al. (2003). The epidemiology of major depressive disorder: Results from the National Comorbidity Survey Replication (NCS-R). *Journal of the American Medical Association, 289*, 3095–3105.

Kopnisky, K.L., Stoff, D.M., & Rausch, D.M. (2004). The effects of psychological variables on the progression of HIV-1 disease. *Brain Behavior and Immunity, 18*, 246-261.

Leserman, J. (2003). HIV disease progression: depression, stress, and possible mechanisms. *Biological Psychiatry, 54*, 295-306.

Lewinsohn, P. M., Seeley, J. R., Roberts, R. E., & Allen, N. B. (1997). Center of Epidemiological Studies Depression Scale (CES-D) as a screening instrument for depression among community-residing older adults. *Psychology & Aging, 12*(2), 277-87.

Lichtenstein, B., Laska, M. & Clair, J. (2002). Chronic sorrow in the HIV-positive patient: Issues of race, gender, and social support. *AIDS Patient Care and STDs, 16*, 27 – 38.

Lyness, J. M., King, D. A., Cox, C., Yoediono, Z, & Caine, E. D. (1999). The importance of subsyndromal depression in older primary care patients: Prevalence and associated functional disability. *Journal of the American Geriatrics Society, 47*, 647-652.

Lyon, D. & Munro, C. (2001). Disease severity and symptoms of depression in Black Americans infected with HIV. *Applied Nursing Research, 14*, 3 – 10.

Maj, M., Jannsen, F., Starace, M., Zaudig, P., Satz, B., Sughondhabirom, M. et al. (1994). WHO neuropsychiatric AIDS study, cross -sectional phase 1. Study design and psychiatric findings. *Archives of General Psychiatry, 51*, 39 – 49.

Mehta, S., Moore, R. D., & Graham, N. M. H. (1997). Potential factors affecting adherence with HIV therapy. *AIDS, 11*, 1665-1670.

Moneyham, L., Sowell, R., Seals, B. & Demi, A. (2000). Depressive symptoms among African American women with HIV disease. *Scholarly Inquiry for Nursing Practice, 14*, 9 – 39.

Noble, R. (2005). Depression in women. *Metabolism, 54*, 49 – 52.

Pence, B.W., Miller, W.C., Whetten, K., Eron, J.J. & Gaynes, B.N. (2006). Prevalence of DSM-IV-defined mood, anxiety, and substance use disorders in an HIV clinic in the Southeastern United States. *Journal of Acquired Immune Deficiency Syndrome, 42*, 298 – 306.

Perry, G.R. (1990). Loneliness and coping among tertiary-level adult cancer patients in the home. *Cancer Nursing, 13*(5), 293-302.

Rabkin, J., Ferrando, S., van Gorp, W., Rieppi, R., McElhiney, M. & Sewell, M. (2000). Relationship among apathy, depression and cognitive impairment in HIV/AIDS. *Journal of Neuropsychiatry and Clinical Neuroscience, 12*, 451 – 457.

Radloff, L.S. (1977). The CES-D scale: A self report depression scale for research in the general population. *Applied Psychological Measurement, 1*, 385-401.

Roberts, R. E., Lewinsohn, P. M., & Seeley, J. R. (1991). Screening for adolescent depression: A comparison of depression scales. *Journal of the American Academy of Child and Adolescent Psychiatry, 30*(1), 58-66.

Singh, N., Squier, C., Sivek, C., Wagener, M., Nguyen, M.H. and Yu, V. (1996). Determinants of compliance with antiretroviral therapy in patients with human immunodeficiency virus: Prospective assessment with implications for enhancing compliance. *AIDS Care, 8*, 261–269.

Tostes, M. A., Chalub, M., and Botega, N. J. (2004). The quality of life of HIV-infected women is associated with psychiatric morbidity. *AIDS Care, 16*, 177-186.

Tryznka, S. L., and Erlen, J. A. (2004). HIV dis*ease susceptibility in women and the barriers to adherence. Medsurg Nursing: Official journal of the Academy of Medical-Surgical Nurses, 13*, 97-104.

U. S. Department of Health and Human Services. (1999). *Mental health: A report of the Surgeon General.* Rockville, MD: U. S. Department of Health and Human Services.

In: Older Adults with HIV
Editors: M. Brennan, S.E. Karpiak et al.

ISBN 978-1-60876-054-1
© 2009 Nova Science Publishers, Inc.

Chapter 4

SUBSTANCE AND ALCOHOL USE

Allison Applebaum and Mark Brennan

Following depression, abuse of or dependence on alcohol and other substances affecting mood or behavior remain one of the principal challenges for people living with HIV. The reported rates of substance use approach 50% in this population (Commerford, Orr, Gular, Reznikoff, & O'Dowd, 1994; Pence et al., 2006; Rabkin et al., 2000). Often substance use appears to be "self-medication" for existing, undiagnosed, or untreated mental health disorders. In turn, substance use can exacerbate these mental health issues. ROAH is one of the first studies to provide a careful inquiry into patterns of substance use among HIV-positive older adults. Studying this behavior in older adults with HIV is crucial. Research consistently shows that substance and alcohol use among persons living with HIV is associated with other mental health issues like depression (Pence et al.), as well as poor adherence to antiretroviral therapy (Chesney, 2000; Ware et al., 2005) and greater risk for HIV infection (Leigh & Stall, 1993; Semaan et al., 2002).

SUBSTANCE USE AMONG ROAH RESPONDENTS

The vast majority of these older adults living with HIV used alcohol (81%) or illicit drugs (84%) in their lifetime. Figure 1 illustrates the proportion of lifetime and current (i.e., past 3 months) use of drugs and alcohol in the ROAH sample. Older adults with HIV were more likely to report using alcohol in their lifetimes or in the past 3 months compared to any other substances except pain killers (i.e., morphine-based pain medications). Nearly three-quarters had a history of using marijuana. The lifetime use of other illicit substances was also high; cocaine (63%), crack (47%), and heroin (44%). More than half of all ROAH participants were in recovery (54%). Thus, the current use of illicit drugs reported was notably less than lifetime use; marijuana (23%), crack (16%), cocaine (15%), and heroin (7%). Very few reported the current use of crystal meth (2%) which has been associated with unsafe sexual practices in men who have sex with men (Nanín, Parsons, Bimbi, Grov, & Brown, 2006). Still, over one-third of the ROAH sample population continues to use illicit substances (37%) or alcohol (38%).

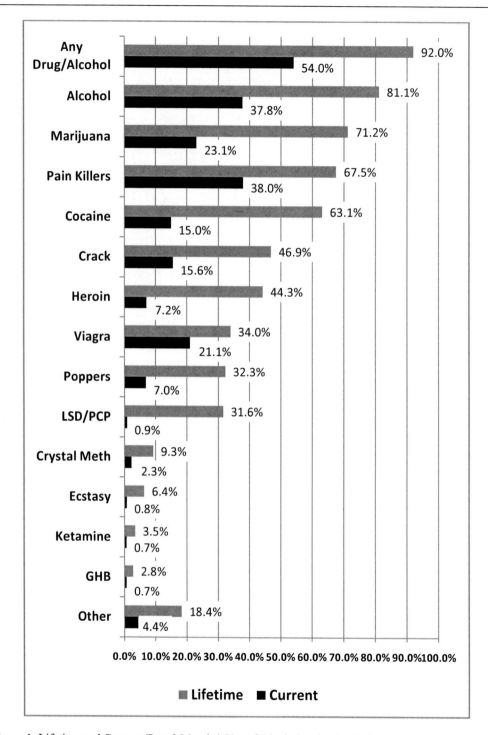

Figure 1. Lifetime and Current (Past 3 Months) Use of Alcohol and Other Substances.

GROUP DIFFERENCES IN SUBSTANCE AND ALCOHOL USE

Reported patterns of substance use are not uniform among the subgroups of people living with HIV. For example, some studies suggest that the rate of alcohol abuse and dependence is particularly high in HIV-positive women (Applebaum et al., 2009; Berg et al., 2004), while heroin and cocaine use is particularly prevalent in men living with HIV (Hartel, Schoenbaum, Lo, & Klein, 2006). There is also evidence that alcohol abuse and use of crack cocaine is more common among African American adults who are HIV-positive (Durvadula, Myers, Mason & Hinkin, 2006; Kang, Goldstein, & Deren, 2006), while Hispanics are more likely to use heroin and/or a heroin-cocaine combination (i.e., speedballs; Kang et al., 2006). Many studies have demonstrated high rates of substance use disorders in gay and bisexual HIV-positive men as well (Ibanez et al., 2005; Parsons et al., 2005). We assessed differences in drug and alcohol use among the primary subgroups of ROAH respondents. Table 1 presents current and lifetime use of drugs and alcohol for ROAH participants according to gender, race/ethnicity, and sexual orientation.

Substance/Alcohol Use and Gender

Men in the ROAH sample reported the highest levels of both current and lifetime drug and alcohol use compared to either older women or transgender persons living with HIV. While there were no significant differences in lifetime use of any illicit substance or alcohol, men were significantly more likely to have used drugs/alcohol in the recent past (57%) compared with either female (47%) or transgender participants (38%). Men reported the highest current use of alcohol (41%) compared to approximately one-third of both transgender persons and women. Men were also significantly more likely to report the lifetime use of marijuana and the current use of marijuana and cocaine relative to women and transgender adults (see Table 1). Although lifetime use of "club drugs," such as poppers, LSD/PCP and crystal meth were significantly higher among men, there were no significant differences in current use, with the exception of poppers. Unlike previous research on younger populations with HIV, the ROAH sample did not show significant gender differences in terms of either alcohol or heroin/cocaine use (Applebaum et al., 2009; Berg et al., Hartel et al., 2006).

Racial/Ethnic Patterns of Substance Use

Older Whites with HIV reported the highest lifetime and current use of alcohol (93% and 54%, respectively), compared to either Blacks (80% and 37%, respectively) or Latinos (77% and 35%, respectively). Whites were also the most likely to report lifetime and current use of a marijuana and cocaine relative to either Latinos or Blacks (see Table 1). However, older Blacks and Latinos were significantly more likely than Whites to report both lifetime and current use of two illicit substances that have become endemic in communities of color, namely, crack and heroin. Blacks were more likely than Latinos to report a lifetime history of crack use (56% and 37%, respectively), but differences in current use were not significant.

Latinos were the most likely to report the current use of heroin (10%), followed by Blacks (6%) and Whites (4%). However, older Whites with HIV were the most likely to report lifetime and current use of club drugs, which likely reflects the high proportion of gay males in this group. However, despite the higher rates of drug use in the White group, older Blacks and Latinos with HIV were significantly more likely to be in recovery (58% and 56%, respectively) compared with their White peers (32%). Overall, ROAH findings on substance use and race/ethnicity replicate findings on younger groups of persons living with HIV, showing that crack and heroin use are sharply elevated among Latinos and Blacks relative to Whites (Durvadula et al., 2006; Kang et al., 2006).

Table 1. Lifetime and Current (within past 3 months) Alcohol and Substance Use by Gender, Race/Ethnicity and Sexual Orientation –Valid Percents

	Gender			Race/Ethnicity			Sexual Orientation	
	Men	Women	Trans-gender	White	Black	Latino	LGBT	Hetero-sexual
Variable	%	%	%	%	%	%	%	%
Drug/Alcohol								
Lifetime	92.9	89.5	100.0	97.3	91.3	90.3	95.1	91.2*
Current	57.2	47.0	37.5*	64.2	52.7	53.1	63.2	50.4*
Alcohol								
Lifetime	82.7	77.2	80.0	93.1	80.4	77.4***	87.5	79.0**
Current	40.7	30.7	33.3*	53.6	36.9	34.6***	48.8	32.9***
Marijuana								
Lifetime	74.4	63.6	66.7**	88.8	69.3	65.9***	80.1	67.0***
Current	26.1	17.0	0.0**	26.5	21.9	24.0	27.4	21.3*
Cocaine								
Lifetime	64.8	59.5	50.0	75.7	62.9	58.6**	63.4	63.7
Current	17.7	9.3	0.0**	9.7	15.1	16.8	13.5	16.5
Crack								
Lifetime	46.0	49.4	33.3	37.1	55.6	36.7***	41.0	49.8*
Current	17.0	12.5	10.0	7.1	17.8	14.7*	13.1	17.0
Heroin								
Lifetime	45.5	41.6	33.3	29.6	46.7	43.9**	28.2	52.4***
Current	8.3	5.0	0.0	3.5	6.3	10.2*	3.8	9.1**
Viagra								
Lifetime	46.9	3.8	10.0***	50.9	31.8	32.0***	42.5	30.0***
Current	29.3	2.3	10.0***	26.1	21.7	19.1	25.1	19.7
Pain Killers								
Lifetime	67.2	67.3	88.9	87.1	64.1	62.5***	71.1	66.1
Current	35.7	43.4	42.9	37.7	35.1	41.8	35.4	39.3
Poppers								
Lifetime	40.1	13.8	20.0***	75.0	22.1	31.3***	65.8	16.5***
Current	9.6	1.1	0.0***	19.3	3.6	7.2***	17.6	1.6***
(table continues)								

	Men	Women	Transgender	White	Black	Latino	LGBT	Heterosexual
LSD/PCP								
Lifetime	36.1	21.4	20.0***	60.9	25.8	28.7***	42.1	26.9***
Current	0.8	1.2	0.0	0.9	0.7	1.4	0.7	0.9
Crystal Meth								
Lifetime	11.3	4.2	10.0**	24.3	5.1	9.8***	11.5	8.1
Current	2.5	1.9	0.0	5.2	0.7	3.8**	3.4	1.9
Ketamine								
Lifetime	4.6	0.8	10.0**	16.5	0.7	3.1***	7.8	1.2***
Current	0.6	0.8	0.0	0.0	0.4	1.0	0.9	0.3
Ecstasy								
Lifetime	7.4	3.8	10.0	24.1	2.9	5.1***	14.2	2.5***
Current	0.6	1.1	0.0	0.9	0.4	1.4	0.7	0.9
GHB								
Lifetime	3.3	1.5	0.0	7.0	1.8	2.4**	4.1	2.3
Current	0.6	0.8	0.0	0.9	0.4	1.0	0.3	0.9

Note. Gender: Men, $n = 640$; Women, $n = 264$; Transgender, $n = 10$; Race/Ethnicity: White, $n = 116$; Black, $n = 455$; Latino, $n = 299$; Sexual Orientation: LGBT, $n = 296$; Heterosexual, $n = 572$.
*$p < .05$, **$p < .01$, ***$p < .001$ Chi-square tests of significance by subgroup.

Substance Use and Sexual Orientation

LGBT respondents were significantly more likely than heterosexuals to have a lifetime history of drug/alcohol use (95% and 91%, respectively), and to have used drugs/alcohol currently (63% and 50%, respectively). Older LGBT persons with HIV reported the highest levels of lifetime and current use of alcohol (88% and 49%, respectively), and marijuana (80% and 27%, respectively). Among heterosexuals, 79% reported a lifetime history of alcohol use, while 33% were current users. With regard to marijuana, 67% of heterosexuals reported lifetime use and 21% reported current use. LGBT older adults with HIV also reported the greatest lifetime and current use of a variety of club drugs compared with heterosexuals (see Table 1). Older heterosexuals with HIV reported significantly higher levels of lifetime substance use for crack and heroin than LGBT indentified-persons. Fifty-percent of heterosexuals reported using crack in their lifetimes as compared with 41% of older LGBTs with HIV, but there was no significant difference in current use. Heterosexuals were also the most likely to report lifetime (52%) and current use (9%) of heroin in comparison with their LGBT peers (28% and 4%, respectively). In line with past research finding heavy rates of substance use disorders among LGBT individuals (Ibanez et al., 2005; Parsons et al., 2005), the overall picture is one of elevated levels of alcohol and substance use by these older adults with HIV relative to their heterosexual peers, Despite these findings, LGBT older adults with HIV were significantly less likely to currently be in recovery (38%) in comparison to heterosexuals (63%).

SUMMARY AND CONCLUSIONS

ROAH's data on substance use, much like the findings reported in Chapter III on mental health, illuminate the co-occurrence of mental health issues and substance use disorders as a major health challenge for older persons living with HIV. The pervasiveness of these issues and their persistence suggests that the limited resources available to address mental health issues among older people with HIV do not appear to be effective. In ROAH, both depressive symptoms and the use of alcohol and illicit substances were highly prevalent.

Substance Use, HIV Prevention, and Management

The abuse of alcohol and other illicit substances among persons living with HIV has significant public health implications since they are highly correlated with unsafe sex practices, and therefore the spread of HIV. The sharing of drug injection equipment (i.e., syringes) can carry HIV and hepatitis. Communities which have adopted needle exchange programs have consistently seen the rates of HIV infection go down and more drug users enroll in addiction treatment programs. While injection drug users who share needles are at higher risk for HIV infection compared to non-injectors, this latter group is also at risk. There is a high correlation between drug use and unsafe sexual activity (Leigh & Stall, 1993; Semaan et al., 2002; Wood et al., 2001), which is the primary means by which HIV was transmitted among older adults in ROAH. For many, the combination of substance use/abuse and sex is a common occurrence as discussed in the Chapter V. Many drug users often trade sex for money to buy drugs. Research indicates that those who abuse substances are most likely to have multiple sexual partners, which increases the risk for both being infected and infecting others with HIV (e.g., Solorio et al., 2008; Surratt, 2007). It must be emphasized that substance use and HIV-risk is not limited to substance users themselves, but also includes their sexual partners who may be unaware of the substance users' behaviors that have increased their risk for HIV prior to the present sexual encounter.

Substance use is also associated with poor adherence to antiretroviral therapy (ARV; Arnsten et al., 2002; Chesney, 2000; Lucas et al., 2002; Ware et al., 2005; Wood et al., 2004). Similar to the effects of depression, the lack of ARV treatment adherence among abusers of alcohol and other substances increases the risk of HIV progressing to full-blown AIDS or developing treatment-resistant strains of the virus. These resistant viruses no longer respond to current HAART regimens and may be transmitted to others, who then find themselves not responding to treatments for HIV.

The need to aggressively address these dual health problems of mental health and substance use/abuse is clear. This is underlined by the New York State Health Foundation's recent establishment in January of 2009 of the first statewide Center of Excellence for the Integration of Care (CEIC). The Center's goal is to transform the system of care for 1.4 million New Yorkers having from both mental health and substance use conditions. This effort illustrates the need to re-examine how these co-occurring issues can best be managed. The CEIC's goal is the integration of mental health and substance use services throughout all phases of the recovery process. This unique effort is based on evidence as well as the challenge of reducing health care costs, especially Medicaid. The outcomes of present substance use and mental health standards of care are not positive in this population. The need to alter the system, if not the standard of care, is clear and beginning to be recognized.

ROAH illustrates that substance use, especially alcohol use, is a dominant health issue for the aging HIV population. Age alone does not provide people with the wisdom or personal coping mechanisms needed to overcome the co-occurrence of substance use and mental illness. Overcoming addictions in this population may be further challenged due to a scarcity of personal and social resources. Better use of existing services that focus on addiction treatment can reduce the risk of transmission of HIV and improve quality of life for people who are HIV positive. The best health outcomes will occur when alcohol and other drug rehabilitation efforts are coordinated with HIV care, including mental health management.

REFERENCES

Applebaum, A., Richardson, M., Brady, S., Brief, D. & Keane, T. (2009). Gender and other psychosocial factors as predictors of adherence to highly active antiretroviral therapy (HAART) in adults with comorbid HIV/AIDS, psychiatric and substance-related disorders. *AIDS and Behavior, 13,* 60 – 65.

Arnsten, J., Demas, P., Grant, R., Gourevitch, M., Farzadegan, H. & Howard, A. (2002). Impact of active drug use on antiretroviral therapy adherence and viral suppression in HIV-infected drug users. *Journal of General Internal Medicine, 17,* 377 – 381.

Berg, M., Mimiaga, M. & Safren, S. (2004). Mental health concerns of HIV-infected gay and bisexual men seeking mental health services: An observational study. *AIDS Patient Care and STDs, 18,* 635 – 643.

Chesney, M. (2000). Factors affecting adherence to antiretroviral therapy. *Clinical Infectious Disease, 30,* S171 – S176.

Commerford, M.C., Orr, D.A., Gular, E., Reznikoff, M. & Dowd, M.A. (1994). Coping and psychological distress in women with HIV/AIDS. *Journal of Community Psychology, 22,* 224-230.

Durvadula, R.S., Myers, H.F., Mason, K. & Hinkin, C. (2006). Relationship between alcohol use/abuse, HIV infection and neuropsychological performance in African American men. *Journal of Clinical and Experimental Neuropsychology, 28,* 383 – 404.

Hartel, D., Schoenbaum, E., Lo, Y. & Klein, R. (2006). Gender differences in illicit substance use among middle-aged drug users with or at risk for HIV infection. *Clinical Infectious Diseases, 43,* 525 – 531.

Ibanez, G.E., Purcell, D.W., Stall, R., Parsons, J.T. & Gomez, C.A. (2005). Sexual risk, substance use, and psychological distress in HIV-positive gay and bisexual men who also inject drugs. *AIDS, 19 (Suppl 1),* S49 – S55.

Kang, S.Y., Goldstein, M.F. & Deren, S. (2006). Health care utilization and risk behaviors among HIV positive minority drug users. *Journal of Health Care for the Poor and Underserved, 17,* 265 – 275.

Leigh, B. & Stall, R. (1993). Substance use and risky sexual behavior for exposure to HIV. Issues in methodology, interpretation and prevention. *American Psychologist, 48,* 1035-1045.

Lichtenstein, B., Laska, M. & Clair, J. (2002). Chronic sorrow in the HIV-positive patient: Issues of race, gender, and social support. *AIDS Patient Care and STDs, 16*, 27 – 38.

Lucas, G., Gebo, K., Chaisson, R. & Moore, R. (2002). Longitudinal assessment of the effects of drug and alcohol abuse on HIV-1 treatment outcomes in an urban clinic. *AIDS, 16*, 767-74.

Nanín, J. E., Parsons, J. T., Bimbi, D. S., Grov, C., & Brown, J. T. (2006). Community reactions to campaigns addressing crystal methamapheatime use among gay and bisexual men in New York City. *Journal of Drug Education, 36*(4), 297-315.

Parsons, J. T., Kutnick, A. H., Halkitis, P. N., Punzalan, J. C. & Carbonari, J. P. (2005). Sexual risk behaviors and substance use among alcohol abusing HIV-positive men who have sex with men. *Journal of Psychoactive Drugs, 37*, 27 – 36.

Pence, B.W., Miller, W.C., Whetten, K., Eron, J.J. & Gaynes, B.N. (2006). Prevalence of DSM-IV-defined mood, anxiety, and substance use disorders in an HIV clinic in the Southeastern United States. *Journal of Acquired Immune Deficiency Syndrome, 42*, 298 – 306.

Rabkin, J., Ferrando, S., van Gorp, W., Rieppi, R., McElhiney, M. & Sewell, M. (2000). Relationship among apathy, depression and cognitive impairment in HIV/AIDS. *Journal of Neuropsychiatry and Clinical Neuroscience, 12*, 451 – 457.

Semaan, S., Des Jarlais, D., Sogolow, E., Johnson, W., Hedges, L., Ramiraz, G. et al. (2002). A meta-analysis of the effect of HIV prevention interventions on the sex behaviors of drug users in the United States. *Journal of Acquired Immune Deficiency Syndromes, 30*, S73-S93.

Solorio, M. R., Rosenthal, D., Milburn, N. G., Weiss, R. E., Batterham, P. J., Gandara, M., & Rotherman-Borus, M. J. (2008). Predictors of sexual risk behaviors among newly homeless youth: A longitudinal study. *Journal of Adolescent Health, 42*(4), 401-9.

Surratt, H. (2007). Sex work in the Caribbean Basin: Patterns of substance use and HIV risk among migrant sex workers in the U.S. Virgin Islands. *AIDS Care, 19*(10), 1274-82.

Ware, N., Wyatt, M. & Tugenberg, T. (2005). Adherence, stereotyping and unequal HIV treatment for active users of illegal drugs. *Social Science and Medicine, 61*, 565 – 576.

Wood, E., Montaner, J., Braitstein, P., Yip, B., Schecter, M., O'Shaughnessy, M., et al. (2004). Elevated rates of antiretroviral treatment discontinuation among HIV-infected injection drug users: Implications for drug policy and public health. *Journal of Acquired Immune Deficiency Syndromes, 37*, 1470 – 1476.

In: Older Adults with HIV
Editors: M. Brennan, S.E. Karpiak et al.

ISBN 978-1-60876-054-1
© 2009 Nova Science Publishers, Inc.

Chapter 5

SEXUAL BEHAVIOR AMONG HIV+ OLDER ADULTS

Sarit A. Golub, Christian Grov, and Julia Tomassilli

The sexual lives of older adults are often minimized, ignored, or even ridiculed. In the media, sexual activity between two older adults is portrayed as infrequent and undesirable. When a comprehensive study of sexual behavior among older adults was published in the *New England Journal of Medicine* in 2007, the high rates of sexual activity were front page news in the *New York Times* and other national newspapers. To accompany their story, MSNBC ran a picture of two older people kissing, and received complaints that the picture was "disgusting" and "nauseating."

In the face of such negative stereotypes and ageist messages about their sexuality, older adults may experience conflict about their sexual desire and expression. On the one hand, older adults may feel embarrassed about a continued interest in sex, and may be left without resources to provide them with information and support about reducing the risks associated with their sexual expression. On the other hand, older adults may be motivated to maintain sexual activity as an expression of youthfulness because a diminished interest in sex may be experienced as an unwelcome indicator of "old age." Older adults may also want to remain sexually active out of a desire to sustain intimacy in both long-term and newly developing relationships.

RISKS OF SEXUAL BEHAVIOR FOR OLDER ADULTS WITH HIV

For older adults who are living with HIV, managing the risks associated with sexual activity remain of the utmost importance. First, HIV-positive older adults who engage in unprotected sex run the risk of spreading the infection to their sexual partners. Participants in ROAH were asked how they thought they became infected with HIV, and over 65% reported that they were infected through either vaginal (38%) or anal (28%) sex. Participants' reported modes of transmission were compared according to the length of time since their diagnosis. As seen in Figure 1, among participants who became infected more than 10 years ago, approximately equal proportions reported being infected through anal sex, vaginal sex, and intravenous drug use (i.e., needle-sharing). Among participants who became infected in the past five years, 49% reported unprotected vaginal sex as the reason they became infected. The increased risk associated with vaginal sex – especially among Black and Latino older adults – will continue to be a critical factor in increasing incidence rates among older adults.

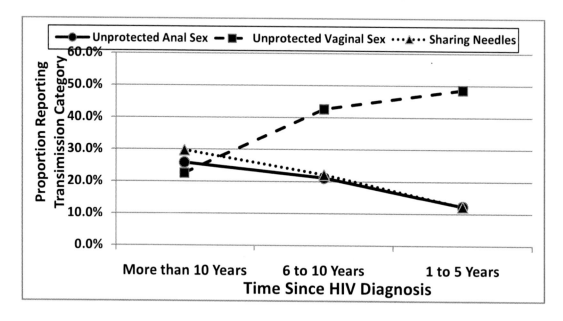

Figure 1. Change in Mode of HIV Transmission by Years since Diagnosis among Older Adults with HIV.

PATTERNS OF SEXUAL BEHAVIOR IN LATE ADULTHOOD

The largest study of sexual behavior among older adults was conducted as part of the National Social Life, Health, and Aging Project (NSHAP; (Lindau et al., 2007). This study interviewed 3005 men and women across the country, aged 57 to 85, and asked questions about their sexual history, sexual difficulties, marital status and relationships, self-related health and other illnesses, and communication with medical providers. In that study, 84% of men and 62% of women ages 57 to 64 reported being sexually active, and 67% of men and 40% of women ages 65 to 74 reported being sexually active. Regardless of age, about 66% of men and women who were sexually active reported having sex at least 2 to 3 times per month.

For these older adults, physical health status did have an impact on sexual activity. Participants who reported being in "good" as opposed to "excellent" health were less likely to report recent sexual activity, and participants who reported "fair" or "poor" health were the least likely to be sexually active. However, among those individuals who reported being sexually active, health status did not seem to affect the type of behavior in which they engaged or the frequency of sexual behavior. Both men and women who reported "poor" health were twice as likely as other participants to report lack of interest in sex, pain during intercourse, and that sex was no longer pleasurable. Older adults with poor health status were most likely to report avoiding sex because of health problems regardless of gender.

In contrast to their level of sexual activity, only 38% of men and 22% of women reported ever having discussed sex with a physician since the age of 50. This finding is supported by other research into physicians' assumptions about sexual behavior and HIV risks among older adults. In one survey of 330 primary care physicians, most (61%) rarely or never discussed HIV or AIDS with patients older than 50 years, and 68% rarely or never discussed HIV risk reduction (Skeist & Keiser, 1997).

SEXUAL BEHAVIOR AMONG OLDER ADULTS WITH HIV

Overview and Demographics

Participants in the ROAH study were asked a series of questions about their sexual behavior in the past three months. Survey items included information about sexual partners, detailed information about specific sexual activities, and condom use. Overall, 50% reported some type of sexual activity in the past three months, and 40% reported engaging in anal or vaginal sex. Self-identified gay and bisexual men were the most likely to report sexual activity (51%), followed by heterosexual men (44%) and women (29%). Similar to HIV-negative older adults, approximately 75% of sexually active ROAH participants reported having sex more than 2 to 3 times per month (see Figure 2). In fact, 57% of sexually active older HIV+ adults reported having sex at least 2 to 3 times per week. Rates of sexual activity did decline with age, with over 50% of participants under age 60 reporting sexual activity, 45% of participants 60 to 64 reporting sexual activity, and 31% of participants 65 and older reporting sexual activity. There were no differences in rates of sexual activity by race/ethnicity. Although only a minority of participants (14%) reported living with a romantic partner, 64% of participants who lived with a partner reported being sexually active, compared to 48% of participants who did not live with a partner.

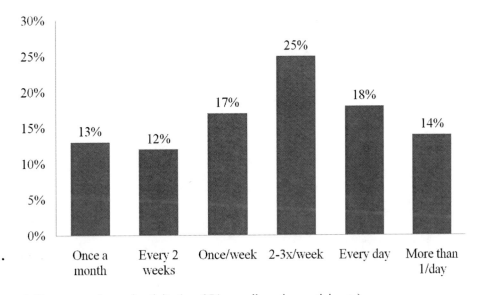

Figure 2. Frequency of sexual activity ($n = 374$ sexually active participants).

Sexual Activity and Health Status

In contrast to some of the findings from the NSHAP study (Lindau et al., 2007), health status did not seem to be associated with sexual behavior patterns for HIV+ older adults in the ROAH study. Sexually active participants did not differ from nonsexually active participants in time since HIV diagnosis, whether or not they had been diagnosed with AIDS, or most recent CD4 count. In addition, sexually active and nonsexually active participants did not differ on self-ratings of physical health, or on more standardized measures of heath-related quality of life (QoL) including physical functioning, cognitive functioning, or pain. Sexually active men did score slightly higher on a QoL measure indicating higher levels of energy and less fatigue compared to their non-sexually active counterparts.

Sexual Risk-Taking

Overall, 41% of sexually active older HIV+ adults reported having unprotected anal or vaginal sex in the past 3 months (see Figure 3). Rates of unprotected sex did not differ significantly by gender or sexual orientation: 47% of sexually active gay/bisexual men reported unprotected sex compared to 47% of women and 38% of heterosexual men. Forty-percent of participants reported exclusively HIV+ partners for anal or vaginal sex, and these rates were highest among women (61%), followed by heterosexual men (36%) and gay/bisexual men (30%).

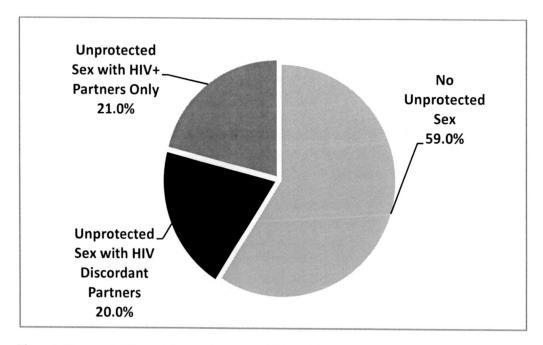

Figure 3. Unprotected Sex and Serosorting among Older Adults with HIV ($n = 374$ sexually active participants)..

Overall, 30% of sexually active older HIV+ adults reported unprotected sex with their HIV+ partners, and 21% reported recent unprotected sex with HIV-negative partners or partners whose HIV-status was unknown. Both heterosexual men and women were more likely to report unprotected sex with HIV+ partners (26% and 21%, respectively) than with their HIV negative or HIV status unknown partners (17% and 10%, respectively). Gay and bisexual men were equally likely to report unprotected sex regardless of partner's HIV status; 35% of sexually active gay/bisexual men reported unprotected sex with HIV+ partners and 35% (i.e., 14% of all gay/bisexual men in the sample) reported unprotected sex with HIV-negative or HIV-status unknown partners. Of the gay or bisexual men who had unprotected sex with their HIV-negative or HIV-status unknown partners, 43% engaged in exclusively receptive sex. Twenty-nine percent of these men engaged in insertive sex only, and 29% engaged in unprotected insertive and receptive sex with HIV-negative or HIV-status unknown partners.

As reported in Chapter IV on substance use, approximately 23% of ROAH participants reported recent drug use. This percentage was slightly higher among sexually active participants; 37% of sexually active participant reported recent drug use. In addition, 24% of participants reported recent drug use in the context of sexual activity. Perhaps most importantly, 40% of participants who reported unprotected sex in the past 3 months also reported recent drug use. This pattern is problematic because researchers have indicated substance use in the context of sexual behavior reduces inhibitions, which in turn reduces the likelihood of HIV status disclosure and protective behaviors (e.g., condom use; Purcell, Moss, Remien, Woods, & Parsons, 2007; Semaan et al., 2002). In the context of sexual behavior, substance-using individuals may be more likely than those who do not use substances to transmit HIV to HIV-negative partners, and to transmit drug-resistant strains of HIV to HIV-positive and negative partners.

Reasons for Unprotected Sex

ROAH subjects were asked the reasons they engaged in unprotected sex. Almost one-third of the subjects who had had sex in the last three months indicated that they would not have unprotected sex under any circumstance (28%). Others indicated the desire for sex (24%) or being with an sexy/attractive partner (18%), their partner's request (32%), being high on drugs (27%), depressive feelings or neediness (19%), and conviction of low risk of STD (14%) as reasons for unprotected sex. Interestingly, the use of erectile-dysfunction (ED) medications was significantly related to being sexually active in the last 3 months (75% of ED medication users were sexually active as compared with 44% of those who did not use these drugs). However, among those who were sexually active, there was no significant association between the use of these drugs and engaging in unprotected sexual intercourse.

AGEISM AS AN HIV RISK FACTOR

Although the number of new infections among individuals over 50 continues to rise steadily, few public health campaigns have been developed to target middle-aged and older adults (Nokes, 1999; Strombeck, 2003). In general, Americans age 50 and older tend to be less knowledgeable about HIV risks (Centers for Disease Control and Prevention, 1994), perceive themselves to be at lower risk for HIV infection (Meah, 1999), and are less likely to be tested for HIV (Ferro & Salit, 1992; Mack & Bland, 1999; Rose, 1995). Even those with known HIV-related risks tend to take fewer steps to reduce these risks, such as condom use, compared to younger adults. In New York City in 2006, 42% of those aged 50 and older who tested positive for HIV also received an AIDS diagnosis. This is compared with only 23% of adults under the age of 50 who learned they have AIDS at the time of their HIV diagnosis. (New York City Department of Health and Mental Hygiene, 2007).

Research suggests several important factors that may delay HIV testing and identification of acute HIV infection among older adults. The first is ageism. Physicians are significantly less likely to discuss HIV-related risks and prevention information with their older patients (Akers, Bernstein, Henderson, Doyle, & Corbie-Smith, 2007). In one survey, both senior center directors and AIDS educators were reluctant to provide HIV prevention information to older adults and reported not seeing any reason to do so (Strombeck & Levy, 1998). The second is the presence of other illnesses that may mask symptoms of early HIV infection. And third, symptoms of HIV infection are often interpreted as signs of normal ageing by both older adults and their medical providers. For these reasons, diagnosis with HIV is often delayed among older adults, increasing their risk of disease progression and opportunities to unknowingly transmit HIV to sex partners prior to learning one's own status.

Many older women think that they have less to worry about with sex after menopause because there is no risk of pregnancy. Ironically, the opposite is true when it comes to HIV (ACRIA, 2007). As women age, the amount of natural vaginal lubricant decreases and the vaginal walls become thinner. These changes put women at greater risk because small cuts and tears are more likely during sex, which give HIV easier access to the bloodstream if the sexual partner is HIV-positive. In general, the physiology of the female body offers HIV easier entry to the bloodstream for women than men during vaginal intercourse. After intercourse, semen stays inside the vagina, unlike vaginal fluid which is easily wiped off the penis. HIV concentration is also greater in semen than in vaginal fluid. Similarly, the receptive partner in anal sex, regardless of gender, is at greater risk of contracting HIV than the inserting partner, because the anal cavity offers more opportunity for HIV to get into the body. The older adult male with HIV may contribute to increased transmission of HIV since the inability to sustain an erection can cause him to either not use a condom, or result in slippage if a condom is used (ACRIA, 2007).

Conclusions: Supporting Healthy Sexual Behavior among HIV+ Older Adults

In addition to concerns about protecting their sexual partners, older adults with HIV must be aware of the risks to their own health associated with co-infection with other sexually transmitted infections (STIs). These can include bacterial infections such as syphilis, gonorrhea, and Chlamydia, or viral infections such as herpes (HSV2), genital warts (HPV), and Hepatitis B or C. HIV-positive individuals with STIs are more infectious to their sexual partners, because the STI draws immune system cells to the infected area (i.e., the genitals). A larger number of immune system cells means a greater number of "hosts" in which HIV can replicate, leading to increased viral burden in semen and vaginal secretions. Second, because the immune systems of HIV-positive individuals are already weakened, STI infections and symptoms can be more severe for HIV-positive persons. And third, fighting STIs may strain an individual's already suppressed immune system, causing their HIV disease to progress more rapidly. For all these reasons, supporting older adults in sexual risk-reduction practices is critical to reducing the number of new HIV infections as well as the morbidity and mortality associated with existing infections.

As the number of older adults living with HIV continues to rise, it will be essential to develop interventions and other supports that will provide them with both information about sexual risks and the skills to reduce these risks effectively. These may include training health care providers to be more aware of sexuality issues among older adults. This could also include training care providers to discuss sexuality with their patients, regardless of age. Though research has indicated care providers may be reluctant to discuss sexuality with their patients, HIV-positive adults may also feel reluctant to bring up sexuality with their providers. Thus, reducing the stigma attached to sexuality among older adults could serve a dual purpose. Older does not mean wiser. Many older adults living with HIV do engage in risky sexual behavior that can spread the virus. Focusing prevention efforts on them and their sexual partners, who are most often peers, is needed.

References

ACRIA: AIDS Community Research Initiative of America. (2008). *Preventing HIV in older adults*. New York: Author.

Akers, A., Bernstein, L., Henderson, S., Doyle, J., & Corbie-Smith, G. (2007). Factors associated with lack of interest in HIV testing in older at-risk women. *Journal of Women's Health, 16* (6), 842-58.

Centers for Disease Control and Prevention. (1994). AIDS Knowledge and attitudes for 1992. *Advance Data, NCHS, 243*, PHS 94-1250.

Ferro, S., & Salit, S. I. (1992). HIV infection inpatients over 55 years of age. *Journal of Acquired Immune Deficiency Syndrome, 5*, 318-353.

Lindau, S. T., Schumm, L. P., Laumann, E. O., Levinson, W., O'Muircheartaigh, C. A., & Waite, L. J. (2007). A study of sexuality and health among older adults in the United States. *N Engl J Med, 357*(8), 762-774.

Mack, K. A., & Bland, S. D. (1999). HIV testing behaviors and attitudes regarding HIV/AIDS of adults aged 50-64. *Gerontologist, 39*, 687-694.

Meah, J. (1999, November 6). *HIV/AIDS prevention in Floridians fifty and older.* Paper presented at the National Association on HIV Over Fifty (NAHOF) Third Annual Living with HIV Into Later Life: Challenges for a New Century Conference, Chicago.

New York City Department of Health and Mental Hygiene. (2007, October). HIV Epidemiology & Field Services Semiannual Report., Vol 2. Retrieved February 23, 2009 on the World Wide Web: http://www.nyc.gov/html/doh/downloads/pdf/dires/dires-2007-report-semi2.pdf

Nokes, K. M. (1999). Are older persons engaging in risk behaviors associated with HIV infection?, *National Associated on HIV Over Fifty (NAHOF) Third Annual Living With HIV Into Later Life: Challenges for a New Century Coference.* Chicago, IL.

Purcell, D. W., Moss, S., Remien, R. H., Woods, W. J., & Parsons, J. T. (2007). Illicit substance use, sexual risk, and HIV-positive gay and bisexual men: Differences by serostatus of casual partners. *AIDS, 19* (Suppl. 1), S37-47.

Rose, M. A. (1995). Knowledge of human immunodeficiency virus and acquired immunodeficiency syndrome, perception of risk, and behaviors among older adults. *Holistic Nursing Practice, 10*, 10-17.

Semaan, S., Des Jarlais, D., Sogolow, E., Johnson, W., Hedges, L., Ramiraz, G. et al. (2002). A meta-analysis of the effect of HIV prevention interventions on the sex behaviors of drug users in the United States. *Journal of Acquired Immune Deficiency Syndromes, 30*, S73-S93.

Skeist, D. J., & Keiser, P. (1997). Human immunodeficiency virus infection in patients older than 50 years: A survey of primary care physicians' beliefs, practices, and knowledge. *Archives of Family Medicine, 6*(3), 289-294.

Strombeck, R. (2003). Finding sex partners on-line: a new high-risk practice among older adults? *J Acquir Immune Defic Syndr, 33 Suppl 2*, S226-228.

Strombeck, R., & Levy, J. A. (1998). Educational strategies and interventions targeting adults age 50 and older for HIV/AIDS prevention. *Research on Aging, 20*, 912-936.

In: Older Adults with HIV
Editors: M. Brennan, S.E. Karpiak et al.

ISBN 978-1-60876-054-1
© 2009 Nova Science Publishers, Inc.

Chapter 6

HIV STIGMA AND DISCLOSURE OF SEROSTATUS

Mark Brennan and Stephen E. Karpiak

Although HIV is treatable and manageable, the disease is chronic and incurable. HIV remains an infection surrounded by fear and myths. HIV stigma finds its roots in the images of the disease (full blown AIDS), coupled with the taboo behaviors of homosexuality and illicit sex, as well as substance use related to HIV infection. Many fear the mere presence of the illness. Others remain unaware or poorly informed about the modes of transmission and risk factors for HIV. Some believe an HIV-positive person's lifestyle led to the infection, and is the result of a moral failure (Reece, Tanner, Karpiak, & Coffey, 2007), or is a punishment for sin (Jue & Lewis, 2001; Lichtenstein, Laska, & Clair, 2002; Raman & Winer, 2002). These myths contribute to the continued negative social attitudes, or stigma, experienced by people living with HIV and significantly inhibits those infected from disclosing their serostatus (i.e., HIV status). HIV stigma is well documented and appears to have increased. One-third of US adults report negative feelings toward HIV-positive persons, including the notion that people with HIV deserved their illness (Herek, Capitanio, & Widaman, 2002). HIV stigma fuels the risk of spreading the virus to others by creating a barrier to HIV testing because the mere thought of receiving a positive test result is psychologically overwhelming.

HIV STIGMA IN ROAH

ROAH data from the Berger HIV Stigma Scale provide evidence that substantial levels of stigma exist among older adults with HIV (Berger, Ferrans, & Lashley, 2001; see Appendix). The measure contains four subscales of *Personalized Stigma* (e.g., Some people who know I have HIV have grown more distant), *Disclosure Concerns* (e.g., In many areas of my life, no one knows that I have HIV), *Negative Self-Image* (e.g., I feel guilty because I have HIV), and *Concern with Public Attitudes* (e.g., People with HIV lose their jobs when their employers find out).

Table 1. Levels of HIV Stigma among Older Adults with HIV

	Total		Disclosure		Personal		Public		Self-Image	
	M	(SD)	M	(SD)	M	(SD)	M	(SD)	M	(SD)
Total Sample	88.9	(22.4)	24.5	(6.1)	38.3	(11.7)	45.3	(12.1)	26.2	(8.0)
	M	(SE)	M	(SE)	M	(SE)	M	(SE)	M	(SE)
Sexual Orientation[a]										
LGBT	81.8	(2.7)	22.2	(0.7)	34.5	(1.4)	42.0	(1.5)	23.6	(1.0)
Heterosexual	91.9	(1.7)	25.3	(0.5)	39.9	(0.9)	46.8	(0.9)	27.1	(0.6)

Note. N=816 for Berger Total Scale. n=812 for Berger Subscales.
[a] For Berger Total Scale $F(1,815) = 10.03$, $p < .005$, Berger Subscales [Sexual Orientation] $F(4,808) = 4.10$, $p < .05$, and [Sexual Orientation X Gender] $F(4,808) = 2.85$, $p < .01$.

The average total Berger Stigma score was 88.9, with a possible range of 40 to 160 (see Table 1). Participants scored higher on items that describe off-putting reactions by others (e.g., "Some people avoid touching me once they know I have HIV") as opposed to items describing internalized negative feelings (e.g., "I feel guilty because I have HIV"). This illustrates that the effects of HIV stigma among these older adults emanates from external sources, rather than negative self-appraisals. They clearly see stigma as an impediment or barrier in engaging their community, family and friends, which is in line with other recent studies of stigma among older adults with HIV (Emlet, 2007a).

GROUP DIFFERENCES IN HIV STIGMA

HIV stigma occurs independent of age, gender, or sexual orientation. This stigma is particularly devastating for those who have contracted the disease but are not members of a high-risk group (Stanley, 1999). For example women living with HIV may experience a more intense HIV stigma in comparison to men. Many women consider HIV to be, "...a dirty disease contracted through dirty needles and dirty sex;" an image that is greatly at odds with society's idealized view of women being "clean and wholesome" (Fisher, 1999). According to Fisher, the disclosure of being HIV positive for women may be "a fate worse than death" because of the social ramifications of disclosure.

In the ROAH sample, perceived HIV stigma varied as a function of both sexual orientation and gender. ROAH finds that the average HIV stigma score was almost 10 points higher in heterosexuals (91.9) as compared to persons who self-identified as LGBT (81.8). The same pattern was observed for each of the four subscales (see Table 1). Findings also indicated that differences between LGBT adults and heterosexuals were also related to gender. As illustrated in Figure 1 with *Disclosure Concern* scores, stigma was significantly greater among heterosexuals when compared with LGBT individuals, and higher among men in comparison to women. However, these differences were significantly more pronounced among heterosexuals as compared with LGBT adults.

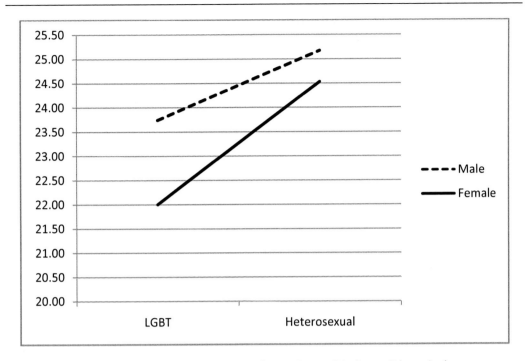

Figure 1. Interaction of Gender and LGBT Orientation on Berger Disclosure Stigma Scale.

DISCLOSURE OF SEROSTATUS

Stigma influences a person's choice not to disclose their HIV status. That concealment leads to a continued HIV epidemic and to the destructive effects on personhood, depression, social isolation and loneliness. What are the social consequences of HIV disclosure? Disclosure of serostatus often results in discrimination that leads to loss of employment, rejection from friends and family, and verbal or physical violence. Although some people can be supportive and accepting, others reject the HIV-positive individual or distance themselves in more subtle ways (Heckman, Kochman, & Sikkema, 2002; Herek et al., 1998).

DISCLOSURE IN ROAH

ROAH participants were asked to indicate their level of disclosure (*All*, *Some*, *A Few*, or *None*) to eight specific groups (see Figure 2). While most ROAH members felt comfortable discussing their HIV status with others, they made careful and specific decisions about whom they told. Not surprisingly, 96% of respondents disclosed their HIV status to healthcare providers. ROAH respondents were more likely to disclose their HIV status to people who were closer to them than casual acquaintances. Thus, ROAH participants were most likely to disclose their HIV status to family members, friends and sex partners (see Figure 2).

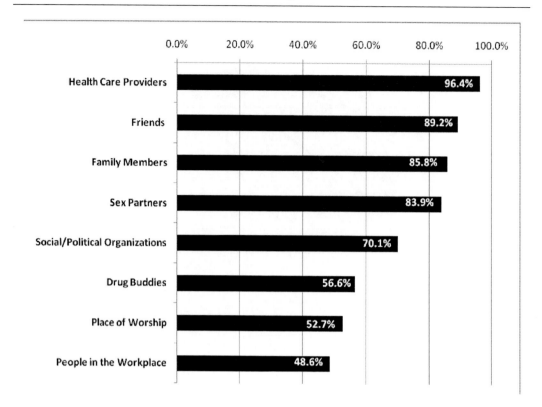

Figure 2. Proportion of ROAH Respondents Disclosing HIV Status to Specific Groups.

Nevertheless, many ROAH members were reluctant to discuss their HIV status, even with people closest to them. While over half (57%) of the participants disclosed their HIV status to *all* of their sexual partners, it is a startling that 16% did not disclose to *any* of their sexual partners. Fewer than half (46%) told all of their biological family members and only one-third (35%) told all of their friends. Similarly, only 30% told all of their drug buddies. Members of social or political organizations, co-workers and people at places of worship were the least likely to have been told of a respondent's HIV serostatus. Twenty-six percent discloses to everyone they knew in social or political organizations. Less than one-quarter (21%) disclosed their HIV status to all of their co-workers. Less than one-fifth (18%) disclosed their HIV status to all the members of their religious congregations.

There were a number of significant differences in HIV disclosure by gender, race/ethnicity, and LGBT orientation that largely parallel differences in perceived HIV stigma discussed earlier.

Differences in Disclosure by Gender

Transgender persons were significantly less likely to disclose to drug buddies (38%), followed by women (47%) in comparison to men (61%). However, in other groups, transgender persons were the most likely to be "out" about their HIV status. While there were no differences in the proportion who had not disclosed to social/political organizations (approximately one-third of each group), transgender persons were the most likely to have disclosed to all of such organizations (40%) relative to either women (30%) or men (24%). Transgender persons were also significantly more likely to disclose their status in the workplace (63%) as compared with either men or women (49% and 47%, respectively).

Differences in Disclosure by Race/Ethnicity

Important differences in willingness to disclose HIV status were associated with the race/ethnicity of the person living with the disease pointing to the cultural overtones of HIV stigma. In general, Whites were the most likely to disclose while Latinos were the least likely to disclose. For older Blacks living with HIV, levels of disclosure depended on the target group. Overall, Whites were significantly more likely to disclose their HIV status to family members (93%) compared to either Blacks or Latinos (approximate 85% of each group). Older Blacks and Latinos were significantly less likely to have disclosed their status to at least one friend (approximately 89% in each group) as compared with older Whites with HIV (98%). Further, nearly one-half of all Whites (47%) had disclosed to all of their friends as compared with about one-third of either Blacks or Latinos.

Older Latinos with HIV were the least likely to disclose to sex partners (81% disclosed), followed by Blacks (85%) in comparison to older Whites (92%). While the proportion of older adults who had disclosed to any health care provider was similar across racial/ethnic groups, Latinos were the least likely to disclose to all of their providers (76%), compared to either Whites or Blacks (89% and 86% respectively). Finally, older Blacks and Latinos were significantly less likely to disclose their serostatus to social/political organizations (66% and 70%, respectively) compared to Whites (80%).

Differences in Disclosure by LGBT Orientation

LGBT adults experience significant stigma as a result of their sexual orientation alone, and are perhaps also less affected than heterosexuals because they belong historically to a high-risk group for contracting HIV. Overall, older LGBT adults in ROAH were more likely to disclose their status compared with their heterosexual peers. Older LGBT adults were more likely to disclose HIV status to family members (89%) as compared with heterosexuals (83%). Similarly, the former group was also significantly more likely to have disclosed to at least one friend (95%) compared with the latter group (87%), and nearly one-half of LGBT adults had disclosed to all of their friends (45%) compared with only 29% of heterosexuals. Older heterosexuals with HIV were significantly less likely to disclose their status to sex partners (83%) as compared with their LGBT peers (87%).

Older LGBT adults with HIV were significantly more likely than heterosexuals to have disclosed their status to all of their health care providers (86% vs. 81%), and less likely to have told only a few or some of their providers (9% vs. 16%) Nearly one-third of heterosexuals had not disclosed to social/political organizations (34%) compared with only 22% of LGBT older adults with HIV. Older LGBT adults with HIV were significantly more likely to have disclosed to all of the people in their workplace (27%) as compared with 19% of heterosexuals, and were also more likely to have told at least one person in this setting (60%) compared with their heterosexual peers (44%).

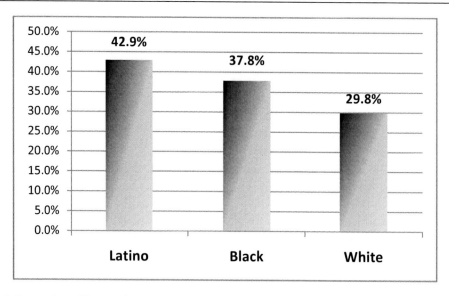

Figure 3. Proportion of Respondents Wanting to Disclose HIV Status to Others by Race/Ethnicity.

REASONS FOR NONDISCLOSURE OF HIV STATUS

Participants were asked if there were people who they would like to tell about their HIV status, but have not yet done so. Almost 40% of ROAH participants reported not disclosing to people they would like to tell about their HIV status. Reflecting the racial/ethnic differences in levels of disclosure, it is not surprising that older Latinos and Blacks with HIV were significantly more likely to indicate that there were others to whom they would like to disclose their status (43% and 38%, respectively), in comparison to their White peers (30%).

Older adults with HIV have many reasons for not disclosing their HIV serostatus to others. In ROAH, these reasons can be grouped into four categories (see Figure 4). While the proportions reporting some of the individual reasons for nondisclosure are small, they do reflect the complex nature of HIV stigma in the lives of this population. The first group describes concerns about the effect of disclosure on others, such as not wanting to worry them (35%), or feeling that they have too many other problems of their own (21%). Other reasons in this domain include others being too young to understand (26%), waiting until they actually become sick to disclose (17%), or their own lack of knowledge about HIV (8%).

The next group pertains to the social consequences of disclosing one's HIV status. These include the fear that if they disclose to someone, that person will disclose to someone else (27%), that others will be afraid of contracting HIV from them (25%), or fears that others will reject them or disclosure will result in losing their job (9% and 8%, respectively). A third group of disclosure concerns involved self-image. ROAH's older adults responded by stating that people would think they were a "bad" person if they disclosed (16%), or that they were a drug user (11%) or gay (8%). Finally, a small but substantial proportion of respondents were afraid of verbal or physical violence if they disclosed; 13% feared the person would become angry, while 6% feared physical injury and 3% feared being killed if their HIV status was revealed.

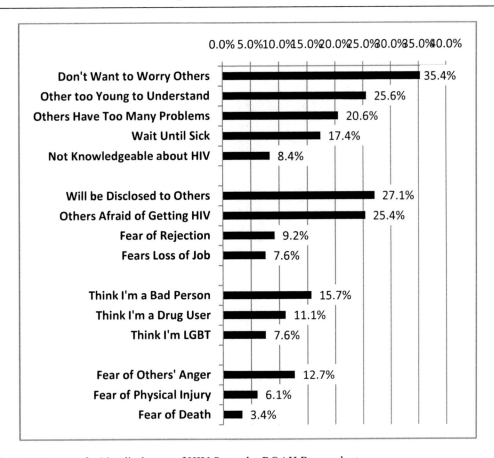

Figure 4. Reasons for Nondisclosure of HIV Status by ROAH Respondents.

SUB-GROUP DIFFERENCES IN REASONS FOR NONDISCLOSURE

Although there were numerous significant differences in levels of HIV status disclosure among the subgroups in the ROAH sample, the reasons for nondisclosure were comparatively constant. The differences that did emerge reflect variations in social and cultural context. For example, older heterosexuals with HIV were significantly more likely to indicate that they did not want to disclose because the person was too young too understand (28%) as compared to their older LGBT peers (20%), reflecting in part the greater likelihood of the former group to have children and grandchildren in their social networks. Furthermore, men were more likely (9%) than either women or transgender older adults living with HIV (5% and 0%, respectively), to report that they did not want to disclose their status because others might think that they were homosexuals, which may reflect the greater social stigma of being a gay men as opposed to being a lesbian. Older heterosexuals living with HIV were significantly more likely to say that they did not want to disclose because others would think they were a drug user (13%) as compared with older LGBT adults (7%), which may reflect the former group's greater infection rates from IV drug use as compared with the latter. Lastly, older LGBT adults living with HIV were significantly more likely to fear physical violence as a result of disclosing their status (8%) as compared with heterosexuals (5%), which may represent a more generalized fear around "gay-bashing" in LGBT communities.

SUMMARY AND CONCLUSIONS

HIV stigma is complex as it operates at many different levels and has both social and psychological aspects, and is more pervasive than most other stigmatizing health conditions, such as blindness. The fear of HIV is so powerful and pervasive that stigma extends beyond those living with HIV/AIDS, to their families and friends, as well as the professionals who provide health and social support services (Reece et al., 2007). Stigma has been part of the dialogue since the beginning of the HIV/AIDS epidemic. There are many factors surrounding stigma including denial, shame, blame, fear, rejection and discrimination, misinformation, and ignorance. HIV stigma has not been adequately investigated or addressed in programs or policies.

The current study replicates previous work on HIV stigma in older adults (Emlet 2006; 2007a; 2007b) using a large urban sample in the Northeast. The experience of stigma for older persons living with HIV is a major source of psychological distress and health risk for these individuals. In ROAH, significant levels of stigma were experienced regardless of race/ethnicity, sexual orientation, or gender. We did find that the experience of stigma may be more intense for older heterosexuals living with HIV, as compared to their LGBT counterparts, suggesting the HIV stigma is more keenly felt among persons who do not belong to what have been considered "high-risk" groups such as gay men (Fisher, 1999; Stanley, 1999). Despite years of epidemiological data indicating the HIV infection moving from gay male communities to heterosexual communities of color, HIV is still largely considered a "pink" disease, primarily affecting homosexuals. Homophobia, particularly in communities of color, fuels the stigma of being HIV positive.

This interlacing of HIV-stigma and homophobia is apparent when we examine patterns of disclosure and reasons for nondisclosure among older adults living with HIV. Greater levels of disclosure were found among persons who identified as LGBT and Whites as opposed to heterosexuals and people of color. Older Blacks and Latinos with HIV were significantly less likely than Whites to disclose their serostatus to friends. This precludes an important source of emotional support for coping and adapting to their illness. More significantly from the standpoint of HIV prevention, older persons of color with HIV and heterosexuals were also significantly less likely than Whites or LGBT individuals to disclose their serostatus to sexual partners, setting the stage for the continued spread of this disease. The same pattern was observed in terms of disclosure to health care providers, putting heterosexual and minority older adults with HIV at greater risk for inferior treatment outcomes.

HIV stigma also has a profound affect on the psychosocial status of older individuals living with HIV disease. HIV stigma exacerbates other types of stigmas faced by many older adults living with HIV, such as ageism, sexism and racism. In older adults with HIV, the stigma involves rejection, stereotyping, fear of contagion, violations of confidentiality, and protective silence (i.e., concealing one's HIV status to avoid negative reactions from others). As discussed in Chapter VII, older adults living with HIV have fragile and truncated social networks resulting in part from withdrawal and rejection because of the stigma associated with serostatus. Consequently, HIV stigma is a key psychosocial problem for older adults with this disease (Emlet, 2006).

It should therefore come as no surprise that HIV stigma is a risk factor for depression in this population (Emlet, 2007b; Flowers, Davis, Hart, Rosengarten, Frankis, & Imrie, 2006; Lichtenstein et al., 2002), including the older adults in the ROAH sample (Brennan, Applebaum, Cantor, Shippy, & Karpiak, 2009). There should be no doubt that interventions are needed to combat HIV and related stigmas in order to improve the quality of life, health, for persons living with this disease. Combating stigma will significantly contribute to the prevention of new infections by removing barriers to HIV-testing and promoting the disclosure of serostatus.

REFERENCES

Berger, B. E., Ferrans, C. E., & Lashley, F. R. (2001). Measuring stigma in people with HIV: Psychometric assessment of the HIV Stigma Scale. *Research in Nursing & Health, 24*, 518-529.

Brennan, M., Applebaum, A., Cantor, M. H., Shippy, R. A., & Karpiak. S. E. (2009). Contributors to depressive symptoms in older women with HIV: Health and psychosocial stressors. In P. Hernandez and S. Alonso (Eds.), *Women and depression,* (pp. 275-310). Hauppauge, NY: Nova Science Publishers.

Emlet, C. A. (2006). "You're awfully old to have *this* disease": Experiences of stigma and ageism in adults 50 years and older living with HIV/AIDS. *Gerontologist, 46*(6), 781-790.

Emlet, C. A. (2007a). Extending the use of the 40-item HIV stigma scale to older adults. An examination of reliability and validity. *Journal of HIV/AIDS and Social Services,6*(3), 43-54.

Emlet, C. A. (2007b). Experiences of stigma in older adults living with HIV/AIDS: A mixed-methods analysis. *AIDS Patient Care, 21*(10), 740-752.

Fisher, M. (1999). From the Advisory Council. *Harvard AIDS Review, 1*. Retrieved January 10, 2008 from the World Wide Web: http://www.aids.harvard.edu/news_ publications/har/spring_1999/spring99-1.html.

Flowers, P., Davis, M., Hart, G., Rosengarten, M., Frankis, J., & Imrie, J. (2006). Diagnosis and stigma and identity amongst HIV positive Black Africans living in the UK. *Psychology and Health, 21*(1), 109-122.

Heckman, T. G., Kochman, A., Sikkema, K. J. (2002). Depressive symptoms in older adults living with HIV disease: Application of the chronic illness quality of life model. *Journal of Mental Health & Aging, 8*(4), 267-279.

Herek G. M., Capitanio, J. P., & Widaman, K. F. (2002). HIV-related stigma and knowledge in the United States: Prevalence and trends, 1991–1999. *American Journal of Public Health, 92*(3), 371-77.

Herek, G.M., Mitnick, L., Burris, S., Chesney, M., Devine, P., Thompson, M., et al. (1998). AIDS and stigma: A conceptual framework and research agenda. *AIDS and Public Policy Journal, 13*(1), 36-47.

Jue, S., & Lewis, S. Y. (2001). Cultural considerations in HIV ethical decision making: A guide for mental health practitioners. In J. R. Anderson and R. L. Barret (Eds.), *Ethics in HIV-related psychotherapy: Clinical decision making in complex cases* (pp. 61-82). Washington, DC: American Psychological Association.

Lichtenstein, B., Laska, M. K., & Clair, J. M. (2002). Chronic sorrow in the HIV-positive patient: Issues of race, gender and social support. *AIDS Patient Care and STDs, 16*(1), 27-38.

Raman, L., & Winer, G. A. (2002). Children's and adults' understanding of illness: Evidence in support of a coexistence model. *Genetic, Social, and General Psychology Monographs, 128*(4), 325-55.

Reece, M., Tanner, A. E., Karpiak, S. E., & Coffey, K. (2007). The impact of HIV-related stigma on HIV care and prevention providers. *Journal of HIV/AIDS and Social Services, 6*(3), 55-73.

Stanley, L. D. (1999). Transforming AIDS: The moral management of stigmatized identity. *Anthropology and Medicine 6*(1): 103-20.

In: Older Adults with HIV
Editors: M. Brennan, S.E. Karpiak et al.

ISBN 978-1-60876-054-1
© 2009 Nova Science Publishers, Inc.

Chapter 7

THE SOCIAL SUPPORT NETWORKS
OF OLDER PEOPLE WITH HIV

Marjorie H. Cantor, Mark Brennan, and Stephen E. Karpiak

Significant resources have been used to understand HIV/AIDS and its effects on individuals, groups, societies and healthcare systems. Few studies have examined the informal social networks of this population which are a critical source of support as a person ages. Even less is known about how these social networks differ as a function of gender, sexual orientation, and race/ethnicity. Research shows that social networks are crucial to both physical and mental well-being for people of all ages, but especially as one grows older and encounters the challenges of managing multiple illnesses, many of which are chronic (Cantor & Brennan, 2000). If the informal caregiving provided by family, friends, and neighbors were replaced by formal caregivers (i.e., paid), the cost would exceed $300 billion annually (National Alliance for Caregiving and AARP, 2004). Will the aging HIV population be able to access informal caregiving and support within their social networks?

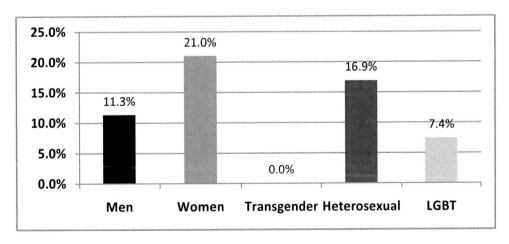

Figure 1. Presence of a Partner or Spouse by Gender and LGBT Orientation among Older Adults with HIV.

It is also important to recognize that the presence of a social network does not guarantee that caregiving and support will be available in times of need. The more germane question is the extent of the *functionality* of the members of the network. Namely, are there people in the social network who are in regular enough contact to conclude that they can be reasonably expected to provide assistance if needed? In two recent large-scale studies of New York City elderly (Cantor & Brennan, 1993; Cantor, Brennan & Shippy, 2004) a functional support element (i.e., person) was defined as someone who was seen at least monthly or talked to at least weekly by phone. This definition was also used in ROAH.

The importance of considering social network functionality is underlined by previous research on the social supports of older adults with HIV. Shippy and Karpiak (2005a; 2005b) found that older adults with HIV had fragile social networks characterized by a reliance on friends, rather than family. Nichols and colleagues (2002) found that older HIV-positive adults did not receive adequate support from their social networks. They reported feelings of isolation, stigmatization, and the inability to cope with the demands of managing their illness, such as keeping medical appointments or adhering to complex treatment regimens. Chesney and colleagues (2003) observed that when social support was available for older men with HIV, they had lower levels of psychological distress and higher levels of well-being.

In the ROAH sample, whose average age is 56 years, 70% live alone (see Chapter II). This proportion is twice that found among the New York City population over 65 where 35% live alone (New York City Department for the Aging, 2009). The vast majority of ROAH participants do not have a living spouse or partner (86%), those who traditionally form the most significant support element in an older adult's social network. Women in the ROAH sample were notably more likely than men to report the presence of a spouse/partner (21% and 11%, respectively). None of the transgender respondents reported having a spouse/partner (see Figure 1). Older heterosexuals with HIV were more than twice as likely as LGBT individuals to report a spouse/partner (17% and 7%, respectively). Taken alone these data describe a population of adults with HIV who have very limited social network resources as they age.

NATURE OF SOCIAL NETWORKS OF ROAH ELDERLY WITH HIV

What kind of informal support networks do the ROAH respondents have? In the following sections we focused on five major elements of social networks: parents, children, siblings, other relatives and friends. For each component, respondents were asked to indicate how often they saw the person and spoke with them by phone. Table 1 shows the proportion of respondents having each of the components of the informal network, and the average number of these network elements, while Table 2 describes the frequency of contact with family and friends.

Table 1. Presence of Social Support Elements and Average Number of Persons in Network by Relationship

	N	*%*	*M*	*SD*
Parent	372	41.2	1.3	0.5
Child	489	54.0	2.9	2.1
Brother or Sister	716	78.7	3.9	3.0
Other Relative	457	50.4	8.5	8.3
Friend	631	69.4	3.9	4.2
Size of Social Network	---	---	9.6	9.2

Note. Percent shown is valid percent. Number of persons in network is based on respondents reporting one or more of such elements.

Parents

Forty-one percent of the ROAH respondents indicated they have a living parent, due in part to the relatively young age of this group. Among older people assistance typically flows from children to parents. However, the presence of a parent can be an important source of help, particularly with respect to emotional support and decision making processes. Seventeen-percent of respondents saw at least one parent on a monthly basis, while 19% saw their parents at least weekly (see Table 2). Levels of telephone contact with parents were also high, with 23% in contact by phone on a daily basis with their parent, and 38% in phone contact on a weekly basis.

Children

As reported in Chapter I, 67% of the sample indicated they were heterosexual, while 24% were homosexual and 9% were bisexual. Having a child is compatible with a variety of sexual orientations, and it is not surprising that slightly over half of the respondents with HIV had at least one living child (54%). Women were significantly more likely to have a child than either male or transgender respondents (i.e., women 73%, men 47%, and transgender 40%). For those who had children, the average number was 2.9. Among men having children, slightly over one-half (52%) see them regularly (i.e., see at least monthly), while among women 74% see their children this frequently. The same pattern is evident regarding regular telephone contact with children; 54% of men have phone contact at least weekly as compared with 80% of women. Heterosexuals were also significantly more likely than LGBT individuals with children to be in regular face-to-face contact (81% and 73%, respectively), but levels of phone contact did not differ.

Siblings and Other Relatives

The majority of respondents reported having one or more siblings (79%). But siblings are less often seen by the respondents compared with parents or children. Only 46% see a sibling with any regularity (see Table 2). One-half of ROAH respondents indicate having at least one relative in the area, but only half of these relatives are in either regular face-to-face or telephone contact. Heterosexuals were significantly more likely to have frequent face-to-face contact with siblings and other relatives (53% and 60%, respectively) as compared with LGBT older adults with HIV (31% and 43%, respectively).They were also more likely (52%) to be in regular phone contact with siblings than the LGBT adults (37%). These significant differences in sibling and relative contact frequency by race/ethnicity reflect the high proportion of gay men in the White ROAH study group as compared to either Blacks or Hispanics. In addition, women were more likely to be in frequent contact with other relatives (i.e., 54% in-person and 79% by phone) as compared with men (52% and 44%, respectively). The infrequency of contact with siblings and other relatives reflects the all too common reports that many families are not welcoming to members who disclose that they are HIV-positive. Issues of stigma, including homophobia, play a role in the relationships among these members of the social network and the older person with HIV (see Chapter VI).

Table 2. Frequency of Contact and Degree of Closeness to Members of the Informal Social Network among Older Adults with HIV

	Parents		Children		Siblings		Other Relatives		Friends	
	N	%	N	%	N	%	N	%	N	%
Face-to-Face Contact										
Daily	45	12.2	91	19.0	52	7.4	32	7.2	233	36.9
Weekly	68	17.0	124	25.8	119	16.9	108	24.3	258	40.9
Monthly	61	16.5	75	15.6	151	21.4	96	21.6	90	14.3
Several Times/Year	63	18.4	81	16.9	127	18.0	104	23.4	40	6.3
Once/Year or Less	133	35.9	109	22.7	255	36.2	104	23.4	10	1.6
Telephone Contact										
Daily	85	23.0	164	33.8	117	16.4	71	15.7	334	52.8
Weekly	141	38.2	154	31.8	215	30.2	151	33.3	222	35.1
Monthly	68	18.4	73	15.1	147	20.6	100	22.1	48	7.6
Several Times/Year	37	10.0	49	10.1	107	15.0	82	18.1	19	3.0
Once/Year or Less	38	10.3	45	9.3	126	17.7	49	10.8	10	1.6

Friends

Like most other older adults, friends are an important component of the informal network of the ROAH respondents. Friends can frequently offer nonjudgmental advice, and some may be available to help with instrumental tasks of daily living as well. Furthermore friends offer the all important opportunities for socialization and network contact so vital to minimizing isolation. Among the ROAH sample, 69% indicated having at least one close friend and the average number of friends was approximately four. But most importantly, it is friends who are seen most frequently and who form the bedrock of the social networks of older ROAH respondents (see Table 2). Transgender respondents were the most likely to report a friend in their network (80%) as compared with men or women (68% and 72%), but reported fewer friends on average 1.0 as compared with 3.4 for the other two groups. Older LGBT adults with HIV were significantly more likely to report having a close friend (82%) as compared with heterosexuals (64%). However, it is important to understand that in ROAH nearly 40% of respondents indicated that at least half of their friends are also HIV-positive, and therefore may not be able to provide assistance if needed. This is similar to the findings of Poindexter and Shippy (2008) who reported that many of the friends in the social networks of older adults with HIV are also HIV-positive. These friendships were largely developed after being diagnosed with HIV, through the process of engaging HIV-support services as part of their health management.

Size of a Network – A Summary

The majority of ROAH respondents have fewer components in their social network than one might expect given the relatively young age of the sample. Less than half have a living parent (41%). Furthermore only 14% indicate they live with a spouse or partner. Children are the linchpin in the social support of older people as they become increasingly frail. But in the ROAH sample just over half (54%) have one or more living children. Although older adults with HIV are more likely to have a sibling (79%) they do not see or talk with them frequently. Furthermore only slightly more than half are in contact with relatives. Friends are the most frequently mentioned component in the informed social networks (69%). Thus, the social networks of the ROAH sample are relatively small in size, rarely involving more than nine or ten persons, and heavily reliant on friends.

FUNCTIONALITY OF SOCIAL SUPPORTS

As noted previously, the critical aspect of a person's social network is not only the size, but whether a person's social network is functional. Does the network include functional members who can provide support when needed? In two large scale studies of New York City elderly, (Cantor, 1979; Cantor & Brennan, 1993) a functional support element was defined as someone who was in contact with sufficient regularity (i.e., seen at least monthly or talked to at least weekly by phone), and could therefore be reasonably expected to provide support if needed.

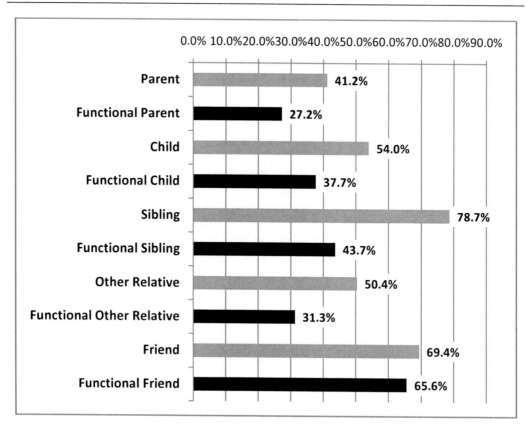

Figure 2. Comparison of social support elements with functional social support elements among older adults with HIV. Functional Elements are those having at least monthly face-to-face contact or weekly telephone contact with respondents.

How many people in the social networks of ROAH participants are functional? In Figure 2, there is a dramatic drop in the availability of functional components when compared to the number in the network. While 41% of respondents have a living parent, only 27% have a functional parent. With respect to children the difference is even more striking; 54% have at least one living child but only 38% of the children are functional and could be expected to provide assistance if needed. Most of the respondents have one or more siblings (79%), but only 44% had a brother or sister who met the criterion of functionality. Similarly, the proportion having functional relatives is only 31%. ROAH data do show that for friends there is parity between having a friend and that friend being functional; 69% of the respondents indicated they had at least one close friend, and 66% had a functional friend. While most ROAH respondents have the rudiments of a social network, these networks are limited or frail. These older adults with HIV are far more reliant on friends than family, the opposite of what is typically seen in older adult populations (Cantor & Brennan, 2000).

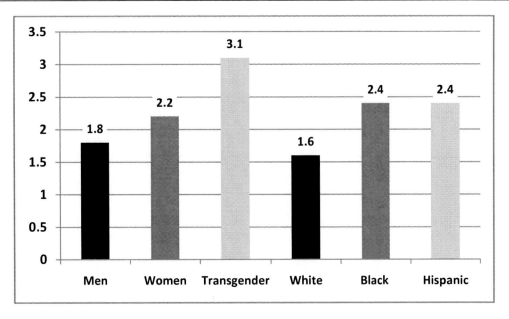

Figure 3. Average number of functional social support elements present by gender and race/ethnicity among older adults with HIV.

THE EFFECTS OF GENDER AND RACE/ETHNICITY ON FUNCTIONAL SOCIAL NETWORK SIZE

Although the size of the social support network is not affected by race/ethnicity or gender the number of functional elements differs (see Figure 3). Whites, who are largely gay and bisexual men, have fewer functional elements (i.e. 1.6 on average) than either Blacks or Hispanics (2.4 and 2.4, respectively). Interestingly, older transgender adults reported the greatest average number of functional element (3.1), followed by women (2.2) and men (1.8).

DEGREE OF CLOSENESS TO NETWORK COMPONENTS

In addition to asking respondents about the members of their networks and the frequently of contact, we were interested in the respondent's sense of emotional closeness to their social networks. Table 3 illustrates how close ROAH respondents felt towards the members of their social networks. Four choices were offered – *very close, somewhat close, not very close*, and *not close at all*. For each of the three major categories the majority reported feeling very close; approximately 64% felt very close to children and friends, and 56% felt very close to their parent. Another large group, ranging from 18% to 31%, indicated they were somewhat close to children, parents and friends. However there was a small group, approximately 17%, who reported they felt not very or not at all close to their primary nuclear family members. These older adults were likely estranged from their parents and children.

Table 3. Feelings of Closeness Towards Members of the Informal Social Network among Older Adults with HIV

	Very Close		Somewhat Close		Not Too Close		Not Close at All	
	N	%	N	%	N	%	N	%
Parents	211	56.4	100	26.7	32	8.6	31	8.3
Children	314	64.6	90	18.5	55	11.3	27	5.6
Siblings	318	44.7	223	31.3	95	13.3	76	10.7
Other Relatives	220	48.4	173	38.0	43	9.5	19	4.2
Friends	406	64.0	198	31.2	28	4.4	2	0.3

The appraisal of family closeness to these members of the social network reflects the attenuated nature of the social resources of many older people with HIV, with less than one-half reporting feeling very close to siblings and other relatives. Sexual orientation affected feelings of closeness to siblings, with heterosexuals more likely to report feeling very close compared to LGBT adults (47% vs. 40%). Furthermore, Whites were only half as likely to report feeling close to other relatives (25%), compared to either Latinos or Blacks (48% and 52%, respectively). This may reflect the high proportion of gay men in the White group who are often disconnected from family for multiple reasons including not having children.

AVAILABILITY AND ADEQUACY OF SOCIAL SUPPORT

To further explore the ability of social network members to meet the needs of adults aging with HIV, a series of questions concerning the receipt of help from kin and friends in two areas were asked; the everyday instrumental tasks of daily living and the provision of emotional support. The questions were posed for each area were as follows: (1) "When you need help with tasks of daily living (i.e. shipping, cleaning etc.) would you say you have someone you could count on to help – all/most of the time, some of the time, only occasionally, not all;" and (2) "During the past year how much more help did you need with these tasks of daily living -- a lot more, some more, a little more, or I got all the help that I needed." A similar set of questions were then asked regarding emotional support, such as someone to talk to or help you make a big decision (see Figure 4).

In Figure 4 several important factors emerge. First the truncated nature of the support networks of the individual living with HIV is evident. Most rely on their friends, a large proportion of who also have HIV/AIDS, which may limit their ability to provide consistent/reliable support or assistance. Because the ROAH sample is best characterized as young-old chronologically, most being in their late 50s and 60s, the full effects of frailty and their need for assistance has yet to be realized. More importantly, the ROAH data underline the powerful affects of stigma and isolation that emerge as a fundamental part of living with HIV/AIDS. We find that only slightly more than 56% of the respondents indicated having someone who can provide instrumental assistance some or all of the time, while the remainder reported that they have someone to help them only occasionally (20%) or not at all

(24%). With respect to someone to talk with or help with emotional situations or decision-making, the picture is slightly improved; 74% have someone to turn to for emotional support at least some of the time. But there is a sizeable minority (11%) who has no one to turn to at all (see Figure 4). Despite the relatively high perceived availability of sources of instrumental and emotional support among ROAH respondents, a high level of unmet need was also evident. Nearly one-third said they needed some more (18%) or a lot more (11%) instrumental help, and the unmet need for emotional support was even greater (42%), with 22% needing some more and 20% needing a lot more assistance. These observations parallel the research of Shippy and Karpiak (2005a; 2005b) which indicated high levels of unmet need for support in this group.

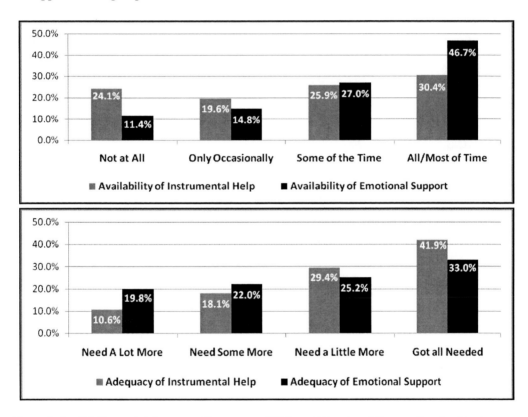

Figure 4. Availability and Adequacy of Instrumental Help and Emotional Support Received in the Previous Year.

DEGREE OF ASSISTANCE RECEIVED

The perceptions of support availability and adequacy discussed above are validated by the findings on the types of assistance they received from both family and friends in terms of instrumental help (e.g., shopping, running errands) and emotional support (e.g., giving advice, talk about a personal matter) among ROAH respondents (see Table 4). The most frequently reported type of instrumental help from family was help with shopping/running errands (38%), while families were least likely to provide help with financial tasks such as money management and paying bills (24%). This pattern was also seen for instrumental help received from friends. The most frequently reported type of emotional support was either having someone to talk to about personal matters or someone to talk to when feeling low, with approximately two-thirds reporting that family or friends provided these supports. The average numbers of types of assistance provided by family and friends was nearly identical (i.e., 2.9 types of assistance from family vs. 2.7 types of help from friends). Older heterosexuals reported significantly greater number of types of help from family members, on average 3.2, as compared with 2.2 among older LGBT adults. This likely reflects the greater involvement with family in the former group as compared with the latter.

Not all social support is positive and beneficial. ROAH asked whether they had encountered negative support from their networks, such as *being reluctant to talk*, *upsetting them or hurting their feelings*, or *refusing to help*. These negative interactions appeared to be equally likely to occur with family and friends. Approximately one-third stated that family or friends had been reluctant to talk or had upset them or hurt their feelings. And one-fifth said that they had been refused help when asked (see Table 4).

Table 4. Receipt of Instrumental Help, Emotional Support, and Negative Support from Family and Friends

		Family		Friends	
		N	%	N	%
Instrumental:	Shop/Run Errands	318	37.8	296	37.1
	Keep House/Prepare Meals	270	32.3	187	23.6
	Take or Drive Places	249	30.0	250	31.6
	Mail/Correspondence	222	26.9	143	18.1
	Manage Money/Pay Bills	198	23.7	130	16.5
Emotional:	Advice on Big Decision	401	48.3	426	54.4
	Talk to when Feeling Low	523	62.5	541	68.2
	Talk about Personal Matters	495	59.0	519	64.9
Negative:	Reluctant to Talk	270	32.6	236	29.7
	Made Upset/Hurt Feelings	296	35.7	269	33.7
	Refused to Help	170	20.6	164	20.6

Note. Proportions shown are valid percents.

COMPARISON WITH OTHER OLDER ADULT POPULATIONS

How do the ROAH older adults with HIV compare with other groups of older people in New York City? Although exact comparison data are not available, two studies provide some valid insights. The study, "Growing Older in New York City in the 1990s" was a representative sample of New Yorkers aged 65 and older (Cantor & Brennan, 1993), while "Caregiving among Older LGBT New Yorkers" used a convenience sample age 50 and older (Cantor, Brennan, & Shippy, 2004). Nearly identical questions on social support were used in these two earlier studies and in ROAH. All studies have ethnic diversity. The citywide study population had a higher proportion of the oldest-old 85 years or more, the very group most dependent on informal support from family, relatives and friends. Two factors emerge when comparing these three studies. The ROAH sample is the youngest and have likely not realized the full impact of old age and associated need for informal assistance. Furthermore, stigma contributes significantly to the life experience of people aging with HIV and older LGBT individuals, but is absent in the older New York City population study.

Table 5 shows the proportion in each sample having the various components of informal networks as well as the average size of the network. Clearly ROAH participants are less likely to have a spouse or partner, thus eliminating an important component of the informal social support network. The truncated nature of the informal support system of the older ROAH sample as compared with a older New Yorkers in general and older LGBT adults clearly emerges. As discussed, while the groups have siblings and other relatives, the older adults with HIV are rarely in contact with them. This results in people aging with HIV having smaller functional networks with fewer children and an increased reliance on friends for support, underscoring the limited nature of the social resources for this aging HIV population.

A similar picture emerges when examining the availability and adequacy of social support. In the two non-HIV groups, the vast majority have persons to rely upon most or some of the time. And all indicate they get all the help they need both for instrumental and emotional assistance (see Table 6). In contrast, the level of support availability and unmet need for help is much higher among ROAH respondents. Thus, not only do the older people with HIV have fragile social networks with reliance primarily on friends and sometimes children, but the ability and or willingness of these members of the social network to provide consistent on-going help appears to be more limited.

Table 5. Comparison of Social Network Components and Size of Social Network: ROAH, Caregiving among Older Lesbian, Gay, Bisexual and Transgender New Yorkers, and Growing Older in New York City in the 1990s

	ROAH	LGBT Caregiving	Growing Older NYC
Spouse or Partner	14%	40%	43%
Parent	41%	32%	NA
Child	54%	20%	77%
Brother or Sister	79%	74%	71%
Other Relative	50%	40%	49%
Friend	69%	93%	39%

One explanation for the limited perceptions of social support sufficiency among older adults with HIV is the fact that many may choose not to disclose their serostatus to family because of the stigma that is associated with the disease (Poindexter & Shippy, 2008). Failure to disclose one's HIV status creates barriers for communication and can contribute to the lack of social support received. Older adults with HIV may be unwilling to ask for help with instrumental tasks of daily living because they do not want to disclose *why* they need assistance. The feelings of isolation and withdrawal from the support network contribute to the high level of unmet emotional need experienced by these people as well. This leaves the real burden on friends. But again many of these friends are also living with HIV/AIDS, leaving open the possibility that they may not be available when the need for assistance arises as they face the increasing challenges of aging with this illness and other ailments. However, as noted by Poindexter and Shippy, these friends living with HIV are optimally positioned to provide emotional support because they are peers. These authors also noted that among older adults living with HIV, having social networks of HIV-positive individuals is experienced as "empowering."

SUMMARY AND CONCLUSION

Research consistently illustrates that presence of family, friends and neighbors positively affects the availability of instrumental and emotional support needed to insure the adequate care of people who are growing older (Cantor & Brennan, 2000). The ROAH data indicate that the aging HIV population will not be able to rely upon typical support networks of partners or spouses, children, or other relatives for needed emotional and instrumental support. At first glance, the data indicates that these older adults have large and diverse social networks. Yet, the majority of participants reported receiving inadequate support. A recent study by Moody and colleagues (2009) found that low education and African American race/ethnicity were both associated with the absence of informal caregivers. Given the substantial proportion of older adults with HIV who fall into these categories along with the social network information obtained in ROAH, it is clear that there will be a large amount of unmet need for caregiving in this population in the near future. Without a functional social support system, older adults with HIV/AIDS may find themselves prematurely relegated to long-term care facilities like nursing homes or reliant on home health care services.

The social network picture presented by the ROAH respondents is troubling. Although the ROAH sample is relatively young with an average age of 56, many already have a level of health comorbidities that reflect a physiological age that is two decades greater than their chronological age (see Chapter II). The absence of spouses and partners is significant, because they serve as the first and primary resource for both instrumental and emotional support to the aging individual. Only 14% of the sample indicated having a spouse/partner and 70% lived alone. For older people, children often provide the largest amount of social support. While many of the ROAH respondents have one or more children, only 38% are functional, and could be expected to provide help when needed. Siblings and other relatives are also rarely classified as functional, even when present. These low levels of contact with family members are particularly noteworthy among ROAH's Black and Latino respondents, in light of the strong cultural emphasis on family ties and reliance on family that are characteristic in communities of color (Cantor & Brennan, 2000). This lack of contact with family members not only suggests that social resources may not be available when needed, but the psychological impact of isolation from family among older Latinos and Blacks living with HIV may be especially devastating.

One must also consider the dynamics between aging and social support. The ability of social support networks to meet the needs of older adults changes across the lifespan. With increasing age, a person's social network becomes smaller due to retirement, illness, relocation, and death of family members and others, while at the same time, the need for such support increases. Cantor's (1979) *Hierarchical Compensatory Model of Social Support* proposes that older adults prefer support from people closest to them, such as partners, spouses and children. When they are not available, older adults seek assistance from other family members, friends, and neighbors in a hierarchical-compensatory manner. When these elements of the informal social network are exhausted or inadequate, the people turn to the system of formal supports, such as community-based organizations or government.

A common process by which older people adapt to infrequent or reduced contact with family is by augmenting their support network by reliance on friends as primary sources of support (Cantor, 1979). For example, research on the social networks of older gay men found that, among men who did not maintain close connections with their family of origin, friends became a 'family-of-choice' assuming many of the emotional ties and legal rights and responsibilities of biological family members (Shippy, Cantor, & Brennan, 2004). Among older LGBT New Yorkers, the lack of a family support has been augmented with an extensive and close-knit network of friends to form a family-of-choice. However, this compensatory replacement of family members has not occurred to the same degree among older New Yorkers living with HIV as seen in ROAH. In addition, the large proportion of HIV–positive friends in the social networks of ROAH respondents suggests that these networks may be further reduced if these friends are not healthy due to increased numbers or severity of age-related illnesses including HIV (Poindexter & Shippy, 2008).

Whether or not the caregiving capacities of the informal support networks of older people living with HIV can be modified is a significant question. Consequently, community-based organizations and aging service providers must assume a larger role and become part of the formal social support system of older persons with HIV. Existing community based formal care services must reach out to these older adults. They are responsible for communicating and providing their services in a safe and non-judgmental supportive environment. The management of HIV/AIDS and age-related comorbidities will have a profound impact on an already challenged health care delivery system. It is likely that the ability to perform instrumental tasks of daily living, such as shopping, cleaning, or getting around outside of the home, will become increasingly more difficult for this population as it ages without formal assistance from long-term care providers, such as a home health aides or assisted living facilities.

One can only anticipate that the demand on the current system will increase due to the growing numbers of individuals aging with HIV, requiring a coherent, comprehensive, and affordable health care delivery system. Older adults living with HIV, who are often low-income and people of color, will "fall through the cracks" and suffer severely. Sadly the aging and often marginalized HIV population encounters barriers to service as a result of continued stigma, coupled with the pervasive ageism that often makes older adults invisible. HIV-related stigma contributes to barriers to accessing the support that might otherwise be provided by religious institutions as well as senior or community centers.

The primary goal of research and treatment during the first two decades of the HIV/AIDS epidemic was to keep people alive and healthy with innovative therapies. In the 1980s and early 90s, it was partners and friends who became the caregivers for those dying from AIDS because they had largely been abandoned by family and stigmatized by society. Today's older HIV population finds itself disconnected from family and again stigmatized by formal institutions. Informal care for persons with HIV is evolving as the need for assistance increases with greater age and comorbidities, as well as the lack of available support. As we traverse the third decade of this epidemic there is a sense of accomplishment for having provided those having HIV with an escape from an early death and a longer life through the use of anti-HIV drugs. But our responsibility does not end here. We must focus on the quality of the life that has been extended to those living with HIV through the medical advances that have made long-term survival with this condition possible, and insure that their needs for social care will be met in the years to come.

REFERENCES

Cantor, M. H. (1979). Neighbors and friends: An overlooked resource in the informal support system. *Research on Aging, 1,* 434-463.

Cantor, M. H., & Brennan, M. (1993). Family and community support systems of older New Yorkers. *Growing older in New York City in the 1990s: A study of changing lifestyles, quality of life, and quality of care, Vol. V.* New York: New York Center for Policy on Aging, New York Community Trust.

Cantor, M. H., & Brennan, M. (2000). *Social care of the elderly: The effects of ethnicity, class, and culture.* New York: Springer.

Cantor, M. H., Brennan, M., & Shippy, R. A. (2004). *Caregiving among older lesbian, gay, bisexual, and transgender New Yorkers.* Final report. Washington, DC: National Gay and Lesbian Task Force Policy Institute.

Chesney, M. A., Chambers, D. B., Taylor, J. M., & Johnson, L. M. (2003). Social support, distress, and well-being in older men living with HIV infection. *Journal of Acquired Immune Deficiency Syndrome, 33,* S185-S193.

Moody, A. L., Morgello, S., Gerits, P., & Byrd, D. (2009). Vulnerabilities and caregiving in an ethnically diverse HIV-infected population. *AIDS and Behavior, 13*(2), 337-47.

National Alliance for Caregiving and AARP (April, 2004). *Caregiving in the U.S.* Bethesda, MD: Author.

New York City Department for the Aging, (2001). *Senior Center Utilization Study,* Report 1. New York: Author.

New York City Department for the Aging. (2009). Quick facts on the elderly in New York City. Retrieved March 20, 2009 from the World Wide Web: http://www. ci.nyc.ny.us/html/dfta/downloads/pdf/quickfacts.pdf .

Nichols, J. E., Speer, D. C., Watson, B. J.,Vergon, T. L., Vallee, C. M., Meah, J. M. (2002). *Aging with HIV: Psychological, social, and health issues.* San Diego, CA: Academic Press.

Poindexter, C., & Shippy, R. A. (2008). Networks of older New Yorkers with HIV: Fragility, resilience and transformation. *AIDS Patient Care and STDs, 22*(9), 723-33.

Shippy, R. A., Cantor, M. H., & Brennan, M. (2004). Social networks of aging gay men. *Journal of Men's Studies 13* (1), 107-120.

Shippy, R. A., & Karpiak, S. E. (2005a). The aging HIV/AIDS population: Fragile social networks. *Aging and Mental Health, 9*(3), 246-54.

Shippy, R.A., & Karpiak, S.E. (2005b). Perceptions of support among older adults with HIV. *Research on Aging, 27*(3), 290-306.

In: Older Adults with HIV   ISBN 978-1-60876-054-1
Editors: M. Brennan, S.E. Karpiak et al.   © 2009 Nova Science Publishers, Inc.

Chapter 8

LONELINESS AMONG OLDER ADULTS WITH HIV

Mark Brennan and Allison Applebaum

While older adults with HIV find themselves living longer lives due to the success of treatment with effective anti-retrovirals, this has not always been accompanied by parallel improvements in their quality of life. For the older adult, social support networks are critical. Yet these support networks are deficient and fragile (see Chapter VII). Many of these older adults lack the core social supports of spouse/partner and children, and have infrequent contact with other family members in the network. The assistance that some receive is largely in the form of emotional support from family and friends, but they perceive that support as being inadequate. Most older adults in ROAH live in communities of color, where cultural norms reinforce the importance of high levels of family interaction and reliance (Cantor & Brennan, 2000), yet such values do not translate into community support for older adults with HIV. What are the psychological consequences of this situation and how does it affect the well-being of this population?

Social isolation resulting from low levels of interaction and engagement with the social network often results in feelings of loneliness. Sometimes loneliness is experienced as a lack of intimacy or commitment to family or friends, or lack of contact or communication with others. Thus, many older adults are increasingly at risk for loneliness as they lose spouses, partners and friends, or become socially isolated due to changing life circumstances such as deteriorating health and frailty (Fees, Martin & Poon, 1999).

LONELINESS IN ROAH

In ROAH, the UCLA Loneliness Scale (Russell, 1996) was used to assess loneliness. Older adults with HIV in the ROAH sample had an average score of 43.9 (SD = 10.6, range 21 to 73). As shown in Figure 1, this is significantly higher in comparison to older adults in general (M = 38.6, SD = 8.7; Adams, Sanders & Auth, 2004).[1] There were no significant

---

[1] $t [1065] = 6.91, p < .001.$

differences in UCLA Loneliness Scale scores in terms of sexual orientation or race/ethnicity, but there were significant differences between men, women and transgender respondents as shown in Figure 2.[2]

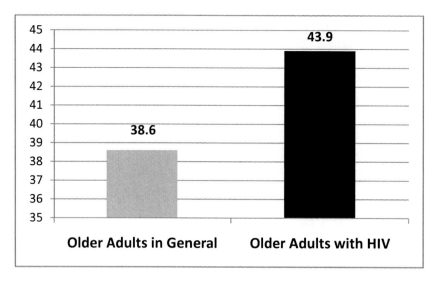

Figure 1. Comparison of UCLA Loneliness Scale Scores between Older Adults with HIV and Community Dwelling Elderly as reported in Adams et al. (2004).

Older transgender people with HIV had the highest levels of loneliness (average = 47.1). Also, older men had significantly higher mean UCLA Loneliness Scale scores than did older women with HIV (44.7 and 41.9, respectively).

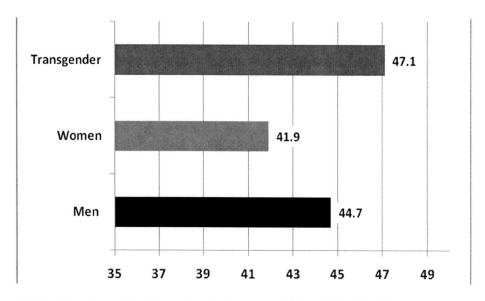

Figure 2. UCLA Loneliness Scale Scores by Gender among Older Adults with HIV.

[2] $F(2, 901) = 7.20, p < .001$.

SUMMARY AND CONCLUSIONS

The high levels of loneliness among adults aging with HIV in the ROAH study has important implications concerning how to provide optimal care, treatment and support for this population. Greater loneliness is correlated with more severe symptoms of HIV infection among women and African American men, who constitute two of the largest subgroups of this population (Heckman, 2006; Mayers, Khoo, & Svartberg, 2002). Loneliness has also been shown to be related to poor treatment outcomes for people living with chronic illnesses like HIV, including heart disease and cancer (Perry, 1990; Sorkin, et al., 2002). Addressing the high levels of loneliness in this population becomes a higher priority as there is accumulating evidence the people aging with HIV are at greater risk for the early onset of age-related chronic illnesses, especially cardiac conditions (see Chapter II).

Loneliness is also related to unhealthy lifestyles choices which include poor diet, lack of exercise, and increased alcohol use (Uchino, Cacioppo & Kiecolt-Glasser, 1996). ROAH also found that these older adults smoke cigarettes at twice the rate of the general population, one of the most significant risk factors for coronary diseases. Such unhealthy lifestyle choices contribute to increased risk for other chronic health problems. Loneliness may also be a factor in transmission of the virus. For example, loneliness is related to greater levels of sexual and drug-use risk behaviors resulting in a greater likelihood of transmitting HIV (Kutz, 2005; Martin, Pryce, & Leeper, 2005; Parsons et al., 2003; Torres & Gore-Felton, 2007).

The most important implication of these high degrees of loneliness among older adults with HIV is for mental health, specifically depression. Loneliness has a strong link to depression in the general population (Adams, Sanders & Auth, 2004), and among people living with HIV (Johnson, Rabkin, Williams, Remien, & Gorman, 2000). Additionally loneliness, and the depression it can cause, may contribute to suicidal ideation (Vance, 2006; Vance, Moneyham, Fordham, & Stuzsick, 2008). In ROAH, there was a strong significant relationship between loneliness and depression ($r = .60$). The high level of loneliness reported by this group of older adults with HIV is likely fueled by stigma and social isolation. In ROAH, HIV stigma is highly and significantly correlated with both loneliness and depression ($r = .53$ and $r = .48$, respectively), consistent with other research on HIV-positive populations (Courteny-Quirk et al., 2006). The powerful role that stigma plays in fostering social isolation and the loneliness that results among people living with HIV, both old and young alike, cannot be ignored.

REFERENCES

Adams, K.B., Sanders, S. & Auth, E.A. (2004). Loneliness and depression in independent living retirement communities: Risk and resilience factors. *Aging and Mental Health, 8*, 475-485.

Cantor, M. H., & Brennan, M. (2000). *Social care of the elderly: The effects of ethnicity, class, and culture.* New York: Springer.

Courteny-Quirk, C., Wolitski, R. J., Parsons, J. T., Gomez, C. A., & Seropositive Urban Men's Study Team. (2006). Is HIV/AIDS stigma dividing the gay community?

Perceptions of HIV-positive men who have sex with men. *AIDS Education & Prevention, 18*(1), 56-67.

Fees, B., Martin, P., Poon, L. W. (1999). A model of loneliness in older adults. *The Journals of Gerontology, 54B*, 231-239.

Heckman, B. D. (2006). Psychosocial differences between whites and African Americans living with HIV/AIDS in rural areas of 13 U.S. states. *Journal of Rural Health, 22*(2), 131-9.

Johnson, J. G., Rabkin, J. G., Williams, J. B., Remien, R. H.,& Gorman, J. M. (2000). Difficulties in interpersonal relationships associated with personality disorders and Axis I disorders: A community-based longitudinal investigation. *Journal of Personality Disorders, 14*(1), 42-56.

Kutz, S. P. (2005). Post-circuit blues: Motivations and consequences of crystal meth use among gay men in Miami. *AIDS & Behavior, 9*(1), 63-72.

Martin, J. I., Pryce, J. G., & Leeper, J. D. (2005). Avoidance coping and HIV risk behavior among gay men. *Health & Social Work, 30*(3), 193-201.

Mayers, A. M., Khoo, S. T., & Svartberg, M. (2002). The Existential Loneliness Questionnaire: Background, development, and preliminary findings. *Journal of Clinical Psychology, 58*(9), 1183-93.

Parsons, J. T., Halkitis, P. N., Wolitski, R. J., Gomez, C. A., & the Seropositive Men's Study Team. (2003). Correlates of sexual risk behaviors among HIV-positive men who have sex with men. *AIDS Education & Prevention, 15*(5), 383-400.

Perry, G.R. (1990). Loneliness and coping among tertiary-level adult cancer patients in the home. *Cancer Nursing, 13*(5), 293-302.

Russell, D.W. (1996). UCLA Loneliness Scale (Version 3): Reliability, validity and factor structure. *Journal of Personality Assessment, 66*(1), 20-40.

Sorkin, D., Rook, K. S. & Lu, J. L. (2002). Loneliness, Lack of Emotional Support, Lack of Companionship, and the Likelihood of Having a Heart Condition in an Elderly Sample. *Annals of Behavioral Medicine, 24*(4), 290-298.

Torres, H. L., & Gore-Felton, C. (2007). Compulsivity, Substance Use, and Loneliness: The Loneliness and Sexual Risk Model (LSRM). *Sexual Addiction & Compulsivity, 14*(1), 63-75.

Uchino, B. N., Cacioppo, J. T. & Kiecolt-Glasser, J. K. (1996). The relationship between social support and physiological processes: A review with emphasis on underlying mechanisms and implications for health. *Psychological Bulletin, 119*(3), 488-531.

Vance, D. E. (2006). The relationship between HIV disclosure and adjustment. *Psychological Reports, 99*, 659-663.

Vance, D. E., Moneyham, L., & Fordham, P., & Stuzick, T. C. (2008). A model of suicidal ideation in adults aging with HIV. *Journal of the Association of Nurses in AIDS Care, 19*(5), 375-84.

In: Older Adults with HIV   ISBN 978-1-60876-054-1
Editors: M. Brennan, S.E. Karpiak et al.   © 2009 Nova Science Publishers, Inc.

Chapter 9

PSYCHOLOGICAL WELL-BEING AMONG OLDER ADULTS WITH HIV

Mark Brennan and Stephen E. Karpiak

The majority of ROAH participants evidenced signs of depressive symptoms (see Chapter III). However, this does not necessarily indicate they are without those psychological resources that enable them to adapt to their illness and life challenges as they age. Given the magnitude of depression among persons with HIV, it is not surprising that most research on psychological functioning has focused on such negative indicators (e.g., Mak et al., 2007), although some have included both positive and negative assessments (e.g., Ramirez-Valles, Fergus, Reisen, Poppen, & Zea, 2005; Rojas, Schlicht, & Hautzinger, 2003). As a result, findings on positive psychological functioning in this population are limited. Because HAART has resulted in HIV becoming a chronic, manageable illness, a balance is needed to assess positive psychological functioning in this population so that we can better understand the full spectrum of their personal resources, and more optimally support adaptation and adjustment as people age with HIV.

THE NATURE OF PSYCHOLOGICAL WELL-BEING

The absence of mental distress does not necessarily imply psychological wellness (Jahoda, 1958; Lawton, 1984). Some have posed the question, "What does it mean to be well psychologically?" (Ryff & Keyes, 1995). Psychological wellness, often referred to as psychological well-being, has many elements such as positive and negative emotional states (e.g., feeling happy or sad), and satisfaction with life (Bradburn, 1969; Diener et al., 1985; Cummins, 1995; 1996; Cummins & Nistico, 2002; Ryff, 1989a). One widely used indicator, life satisfaction ratings, presents a person's overall perception of their well-being. This perception is comprised of many components including material well-being, health, and emotional well-being (Cummins, 1996). The relative importance of these categories varies from person to person so that what one person finds satisfying may be different from another person. Life satisfaction has been a frequent topic of research and there is a substantial amount of comparison data available.

Cummins and Nistico (2002) proposed that life satisfaction ratings depend upon a rich psychological process that promotes a positive view of life, including a positive sense of self-worth, the ability to control life's situations, and feelings of optimism. For example, spinal cord injury patients may maintain optimistic, and sometimes unrealistic, attitudes about their ability to control their recovery through personal effort or dedication, despite having sustained a major physical and life-altering trauma. These coping mechanisms develop as ways for people to best manage their lives even in the face of stark adversity, and still maintain some sense of personal integrity. Adaptational processes involving this type of coping could prove to be very important for older adults living with HIV, protecting them from the negative psychosocial consequences of their illness, such as depression, anxiety, loneliness and stigma.

LIFE SATISFACTION IN ROAH

In ROAH life satisfaction was assessed by asking, "All things considered, how satisfied are you with your life these days?" Respondents indicated a value between 0 and 10, with higher scores indicating greater life satisfaction. Scores on this item averaged 7.3 ($SD = 1.9$), which was above the midpoint of five on the scale, indicating relatively high levels of life satisfaction in the ROAH sample. There were no significant differences on life satisfaction when comparing gender or sexual orientation. However, as seen in Figure 1, Blacks and Latinos had significantly higher levels of life satisfaction ($M = 7.5$, $SD = 1.7$, and $M = 7.3$, $SD = 1.9$, respectively) when compared to Whites ($M = 6.4$, $SD = 2.4$)[1].

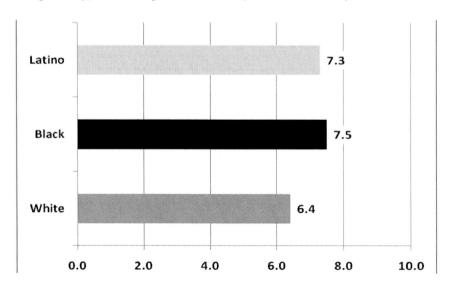

Figure 1. Life Satisfaction Ratings by Race/Ethnicity.

_____

[1] $F(2,801) = 3.82, p = .022$

RYFF'S SCALES OF PSYCHOLOGICAL WELL-BEING

Carol Ryff and colleagues have conducted pioneering research on psychological well-being in recent decades with the development of a 6-factor model of psychological well-being (*Autonomy, Environmental Mastery, Personal Growth, Positive Relations with Others, Purpose in Life,* and *Self-Acceptance*; Ryff, 1989a; 1989b; 1989c). These facets of well-being are often identified as elements of successful aging and considered essential to life quality in both theoretical work and in studies of the general population (Rowe & Kahn, 1998; Ryff, 1989b; 1989c).

In ROAH the 9-item versions of Ryff's *Scales of Psychological Well-Being* (Ryff, 1989c) were used to assess the personal resources and psychological functioning of older adults with HIV. These scales have a range of 9 to 54, with higher scores indicating greater well-being. Each scale has a midpoint of 31.5. ROAH is the first study of an HIV-positive population in which these scales were used. Findings on the Ryff Scales are presented here with a brief description of each domain to provide a context for these assessments.

Autonomy

Autonomous people are self-determining and independent, able to resist social pressures to think and act in certain ways. They judge themselves by their own set of standards and regulate their behavior based upon these standards. Most of the ROAH participants scored nearly 10 points higher than the midpoint of the scale, indicating that most of these older adults have a clear sense of identity and independence (see Table 1).

Table 1. Multivariate Tests of Average Scores and Significant Group Differences on Ryff's Scales of Psychological Well-being

	Autonomy		Mastery		Personal		Positive		Purpose		Acceptance	
	M	*(SD)*	*M*	*(SD)*	*M*	*(SD)*	*M*	*(SD)*	*M*	*(SD)*	*M*	*(SD)*
Total	41.4	(7.4)	39.0	(8.2)	41.1	(8.0)	39.3	(8.6)	38.1	(9.0)	38.4	(8.5)
Race /Ethnicity[a]												
White	41.8	(7.6)	*36.3*	*(9.7)*	**42.7**	**(8.0)**	*38.3*	*(9.0)*	38.7	(8.4)	*36.5*	*(10.7)*
Black	**42.2**	**(7.2)**	**40.1**	**(7.7)**	41.8	(7.5)	**40.1**	**(8.4)**	**40.3**	**(8.1)**	**39.0**	**(8.0)**
Hispanic	*40.2*	*(7.6)*	38.4	(8.1)	*39.3*	*(8.5)*	*38.4*	*(8.7)*	*38.1*	*(9.0)*	38.2	(8.3)
Sexual Orientation[b]												
Heterosexual	*41.0*	*(7.4)*	**39.1**	**(7.7)**	*40.4*	*(8.0)*	*39.1*	*(8.3)*	39.3	(8.2)	*38.2*	*(8.0)*
LGBT	**42.2**	**(7.5)**	*38.8*	*(9.3)*	**42.3**	**(8.0)**	**39.7**	**(9.2)**	39.3	(9.1)	**38.7**	**(9.5)**

Note. Listwise *N* = 783. *Autonomy* – Autonomy Scale; *Mastery* – Environmental Mastery; *Personal* – Personal Growth; *Positive* – Positive Relations with Others; *Purpose* – Purpose and Meaning in Life; *Acceptance*–Self Acceptance. Highest subgroup mean scores are **bolded** and lowest are *italicized.*

[a] Multivariate $F(12, 771) = 2.14, p < .01.$

[b] Multivariate $F(6, 777) = 2.64, p < .02.$

Environmental Mastery

A person who scores high on this scale is able to adapt to or create a comfortable environment that is suitable to his or her personal needs and values. This particular domain of well-being is integral to an older HIV-positive adult's ability to live in a society that discriminates against people with HIV and being older. ROAH participants had average scores that were 9 points above the scale's midpoint, suggesting that many feel a sense of competence in dealing with the world around them.

Personal Growth

Older adults with HIV who are open to new experiences and see improvement in their attitudes and behaviors over time will be more likely to adhere to treatment regimens and actively seek new information about their illness. These people can become more self-aware and realize their potential, further reinforcing positive psychosocial and physiological health. The average score for Personal Growth was one of the highest in ROAH with average scores 10 points greater than the midpoint, indicating that this group of older adults with HIV is receptive to new opportunities for personal development.

Positive Relations with others

An older HIV-positive adult who has strong relationships with others is concerned with others' welfare and is capable of empathy, affection and intimacy. That person can develop mutually beneficial relationships, which provide needed instrumental and emotional support. ROAH participants' average score on this scale was 39.3 which was 8 points above the midpoint. This finding is encouraging given the burden of social isolation and loneliness experienced by many of the older adults in ROAH (see Chapters VII and VIII, respectively), because it reflects a psychological capacity to form and nurture relationships vital to successful aging.

Purpose in Life

A sense of meaning for one's past and present life experiences can assist an older adult with HIV in creating personal goals and objectives for living that result in positive adaptation to their illness. The person may be less likely to feel victimized and, therefore, more proactive in seeking information and assistance with their illness. The average score among older adults with HIV was 7 points above the scale midpoint, indicating a relative strength in this area. This parallels other findings in ROAH which indicated that purpose in life is a dominant aspect of spirituality in this population (see Chapter X).

Self-Acceptance

A self-accepting person possesses a positive attitude, acknowledges and accepts both good and bad aspects of him- or herself, and feels positive about his or her past life. Although this scale had one of the lowest averages of the six scales (M = 38.4), it was still approximately 7 points above the midpoint. Given the frequently hostile attitude of society toward people living with HIV as evidenced by the high levels of perceived stigma in the ROAH sample (see Chapter VI), it is important for them to achieve a high level of self-acceptance in order to sustain a positive outlook on life.

GROUP DIFFERENCES IN PSYCHOLOGICAL WELL-BEING

In ROAH, a number of significant differences emerged using the Ryff Scales (1989c) by gender, race/ethnicity, and sexual orientation (see Table 1). Older Blacks with HIV had the highest average levels of well-being on five of the six indicators, except for *Personal Growth* on which Whites had the highest average score. Overall, this suggests a significant level of psychological hardiness among older Blacks with HIV. This might be in part a reflection of their having confronted racism throughout their lives. In a similar pattern, older LGBT individuals with HIV had significantly higher scores on five of the six dimensions compared to heterosexuals, except for *Environmental Mastery*. As was the case with Blacks, people who are LGBT endure considerable harassment and discrimination, which may have contributed to a higher level of psychological hardiness as they adjusted to living with HIV.

There were also complex differences between men and women on these assessments that varied depending upon sexual orientation.[2] Using the *Autonomy* scale as an example (see Figure 2), older LGBT adults with HIV scored higher then heterosexuals on well-being. In addition, although women had higher well-being scores than men overall, this difference was not as evident in the LGBT group compared to heterosexuals. Furthermore, the pattern of differences indicates that when psychological functioning among older people with HIV is examined by gender and sexual orientation, older Lesbians living with HIV emerge with the highest levels of psychological well-being, followed by gay men, heterosexual women, and lastly, heterosexual men. Past research on group differences (e.g., age, race/ethnicity, or sexual orientation) in psychological well-being using the Ryff scales is limited. The only reliable previously reported differences on these measures is between men and women on *Positive Relations with Others* (Ryff, 1989c), where women's higher self-rankings in this domain likely reflect their tendency to place a higher value on interpersonal relationships when compared to men.

---

[2] F (6,777) = 2.19, $p <. 05$

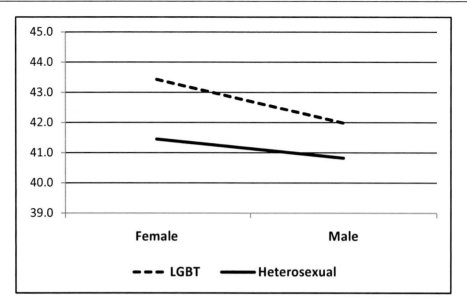

Figure 2. Effects of LGBT Orientation and Gender on Ryff's Scales of Psychological Well-being: Autonomy Scale.

DIFFERENCES IN LEVELS OF WELL-BEING BASED ON HIV STATUS

How does the ROAH sample compare to the general population on psychological well-being? Differences in well-being by HIV status were examined using comparative data reported by Ryff and Keyes (1995) from a sample of 1,108 adults 25 and older in the U.S. with an average age of 46. This study used the 3-item version of the Ryff scales, in contrast to the 9-item version used in ROAH. Data reported from each sample was standardized to the same metric before analysis (see Table 2). While there are obvious limits to this approach, it does provide a preliminary assessment of how psychological functioning may differ between people with HIV and those who do not have the virus. The ROAH sample had significantly lower average scores on the six dimensions of well-being when compared to the Ryff and Keyes sample. This suggests the older adults with HIV are at a disadvantage in the area of positive psychological functioning. This was not unexpected given the psychosocial impact of HIV-stigma, which has been found to predict poorer psychological well-being in younger groups of the HIV population (Mak et al., 2007). Lower well-being is also related to other life circumstances (e.g., low income) and the burden of depressive symptoms experienced by many older adults with HIV.

CONCLUSIONS

ROAH's findings on psychological well-being create a multifaceted picture for adults aging with HIV in the context of a society that is often hostile. Mak and colleagues (2007) noted the connection between HIV-stigma and well-being, and contend that people living with HIV may experience lower levels of psychological well-being than those who are not infected because of the pervasiveness of HIV-stigma. Indeed, a comparison of the Ryff measures between a large national sample of community dwelling adults and ROAH found lower levels of well-being in the HIV-positive group. ROAH also finds high levels of perceived stigma in this population (see Chapter VI). These internalized perceptions indicate that many challenges still exist for this group in terms of maintaining and improving their psychological wellness as they cope with the dual challenges of living with HIV and growing older.

Table 2. Comparison of Scores on Ryff's Scales of Psychological Well-being between ROAH and National Probability Sample[a]

	Autonomy		Mastery		Personal		Positive		Purpose		Acceptance	
	M	*(SD)*	*M*	*(SD)*	*M*	*(SD)*	*M*	*(SD)*	*M*	*(SD)*	*M*	*(SD)*
ROAH												
Raw	41.4	(7.4)	39.0	(8.2)	41.1	(8.0)	39.3	(8.6)	38.1	(9.0)	38.4	(8.5)
Standardized	4.6	(0.8)	4.3	(0.9)	4.6	(0.9)	4.4	(1.0)	4.2	(1.0)	4.3	(0.9)
National Sample[a]												
Raw	15.2	(2.6)	14.9	(2.8)	15.7	(2.5)	14.8	(3.2)	14.4	(3.2)	14.6	(3.1)
Standardized	5.1	(0.9)	5.0	(0.9)	5.2	(0.8)	4.9	(1.1)	4.8	(1.1)	4.9	(1.0)
t-value ($df = 1,704$)	12.0^{***}		16.0^{***}		14.6^{***}		9.8^{***}		11.7^{***}		12.9^{***}	

Note. Listwise $N = 783$. *Autonomy* – Autonomy Scale; *Mastery* – Environmental Mastery; *Personal* – Personal Growth; *Positive* – Positive Relations with Others; *Purpose* – Purpose and Meaning in Life; *Acceptance* – Self Acceptance.
[a] National probability sample and data reported in Ryff & Keyes (1995). Listwise $N = 923$.

The findings regarding higher levels of well-being related to race/ethnicity and LGBT orientation are of particular interest and suggest a certain psychological hardiness in some segments of this population. Older people of color with HIV had higher life satisfaction ratings compared to Whites, while Blacks tended to have the highest levels of psychological well-being on the six-factor measure. Similarly, older LGBT adults with HIV had higher levels of well-being than their heterosexual counterparts. Both people of color and LGBT individuals encounter considerable stigma, discrimination, and prejudice in our society independent of their HIV status. Developing coping mechanisms in order to confront that adversity may have given them enhanced psychological resources. Those resources may have allowed them to better adjust to living with HIV and its associated stigma. This type of psychological hardiness may be crucial for older adults living with HIV to achieve successful aging and enjoy an optimal quality-of-life as their years advance (Vance, Burrage, Couch, & Raper, 2008).

REFERENCES

Bradburn, N. M. (1969). *The structure of psychological well-being*. Chicago: Aldine Publishing Co.

Cummins, R. A. (1995). On the trail of the gold standard for subjective well-being. *Social Indicators Research, 35*, 179-200.

Cummins, R. A. (1996). The domains of life satisfaction: An attempt to order chaos. *Social Indicators Research, 38,* 303-28.

Cummins, R. A., & Nistico, H. (2002). Maintaining life satisfaction: The role of positive cognitive bias. *Journal of Happiness Studies, 3,* 37-69.

Diener, E., & Larson, R. J., Levine, S., & Emmons, R. A. (1985). Intensity and frequency: Dimensions underlying positive and negative affect. *Journal of Personality and Social Psychology, 48,* 1253-65.

Jahoda, M. (1958). Current *concepts of positive mental health.* New York: Basic Books.

Kennedy, C. A. (1995). Gender differences in HIV-related psychological distress in heterosexual couples. *AIDS Care, 7*(1), 33-8.

Lawton, M. P. (1984). The varieties of well-being. In C. Z. Malatesta & C. E. Izard (Eds.), *Emotion in adult development.* Beverly Hills, CA: Sage.

Mak, W. W. S., Cheung, R. Y. M., Law, R. W., Woo, J., Li, P. C. K., & Chung, R. Y. W. (2007). Examining attribution model of self-stigma on social support and psychological well-being among people with HIV +/AIDS. *Social Science & Medicine, 64*(8), 1549-60.

Ramirez-Valles, J., Fergus, S., Reisen, C. A., Poppen, P. J.,& Zea, M. C. (2005). Confronting stigma: Community involvement and psychological well-being among HIV-positive Latino gay men. *Hispanic Journal of Behavioral Sciences, 27*(1), 101-20.

Rojas, R., Schlicht, W., & Hautzinger, M. (2003). Effects of exercise training on quality of life, psychological well-being, immune status, and cardiopulmonary fitness in an HIV-1 positive population. *Journal of Sport & Exercise Psychology, 25,* 440-56.

Rowe, J. W., & Kahn, R. L. (1998). *Successful aging.* New York: Pantheon Books.

Ryff, C. D. (1989a). Beyond Ponce De Leon and life satisfaction: New directions in quest of successful ageing. *International Journal of Behavioral Development, 12*(1), 35-55.

Ryff, C. D. (1989b). In the eye of the beholder: Views of psychological well-being among middle-age and older adults. *Psychology & Aging, 4*(2), 195-210.

Ryff, C.D. (1989c). Happiness is everything, or is it? Explorations on the meaning of psychological well-being. *Journal of Personality and Social Psychology, 57,* 1069-1081.

Ryff, C. D. & Keyes, K. L. M. (1995). The structure of psychological well-being revisited. *Journal of Personality and Social Psychology, 69*(4), 719-727.

Vance, D. E., Burrage, J. Jr., Couch, A., & Raper, J. (2008). Promoting successful aging with HIV through hardiness: Implications for nursing practice and research. *Journal of Gerontological Nursing, 34*(6), 22-9.

In: Older Adults with HIV
Editors: M. Brennan, S.E. Karpiak et al.
ISBN 978-1-60876-054-1
© 2009 Nova Science Publishers, Inc.

Chapter 10

RELIGIOUSNESS AND SPIRITUALITY

Mark Brennan

Religion and spirituality can be critical personal resources for older adults as they adapt to a chronic illness and the challenges of aging. Religion and spirituality are overlapping concepts, but with distinct differences. Religiousness is an engagement with a belief system associated with a particular faith or creed (Moberg, 1967; Pargament, 1997). Definitions of spirituality include feelings of existential well-being involving transcendence over one's circumstances, feeling purpose and meaning in life, a sense of inner-integration, and connectedness with others (Howden, 1992; Lindgren & Coursey, 1995; Moberg, 1967). Further, religious and faith-based institutions are an important source of support and comfort. They are often pivotal cultural elements in the community-life of many racial and ethnic groups, particularly Latinos and African Americans (Espinosa, 2008; Lewis & Trulear, 2008-09).

Religion and spirituality can be a vital personal resource for people living with HIV. In one study 65% considered religion and 85% considered spirituality to have some level of importance in their lives (Lorenz, Hays, Shapiro, Cleary, Asch, & Wegner, 2005). While research has examined the function of religion and spirituality among persons living with HIV, there are few studies that specifically assess older adults with HIV and spirituality. People living with HIV, including older adults, experience a strong need for meaning and hope. Why? Spirituality and religious beliefs and practices can assist in helping them to cope and adjust to challenges of living with this chronic yet life-threatening illness (Dunphy, 1987; Gehr, 2002; Kalichman, 1998), as well as other circumstances that are viewed as unfair or without any sense of balance, such as HIV stigma, social isolation, or other problems. Siegel and Schrimshaw (2002) reported that among older persons with HIV (50 to 68 years), religious/spiritual beliefs and practices provided benefit that included emotional and spiritual support, reduced anxiety, and increased feelings of self-acceptance. Spirituality and religiousness are catalysts for people with HIV. These personal resources allow them to strengthen their connections with others and permit the activation of vitally important social support which are crucial in helping them adapt to an often arduous condition (Heinrich, 2003; Kendall, 1994; Siegel & Schrimshaw).

RELIGIOUS AFFILIATION AND PARTICIPATION

In ROAH, the majority reported Christian religious affiliations of Protestant and Catholic (42% and 34%, respectively). Smaller proportions reported being Muslim or Jewish (6% and 2%, respectively), while 12% reported some "other" affiliation. Smaller proportions identified as being Hindu (0.2%) or Buddhist (2%), or atheists (2%).

Because there are interrelationships between culture and religion, it is not surprising that religious affiliation[1] varied significantly as a function of gender, race/ethnicity, and sexual orientation. Older women with HIV were more likely to be Protestant (53%), as compared with either men or transgender adults (37% and 13%, respectively). While men were more likely to report being Muslim (8%) compared to both women and transgender older adults with HIV (3% and 0%, respectively). Latinos were predominantly Catholic (59%), followed by Whites (42%) and Blacks (15%). In contrast, Blacks were the most likely to report being Protestant or Muslim (see Figure 1). Considering sexual orientation, heterosexuals were significantly more likely than LGBT older adults with HIV to report being Protestant (47% and 29%, respectively) or Muslim (10% and 1%, respectively.) LGBT older adults were the more likely to identify as Jewish (6%), as compared with 1% of heterosexuals.

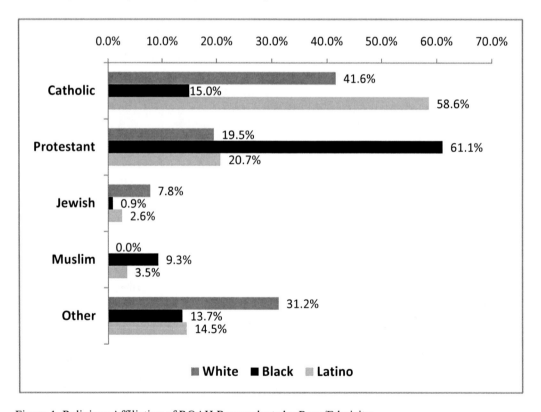

Figure 1. Religious Affiliation of ROAH Respondents by Race/Ethnicity.

---

[1] For these analyses, religious affiliation was collapsed into five groups; Catholic, Protestant, Muslim, Jewish, and all others (i.e., Hindu, Buddhist, Atheist, and Other).

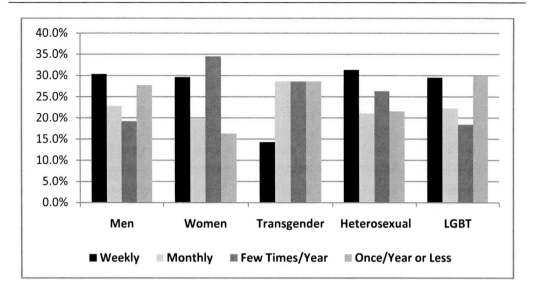

Figure 2. Frequency of Religious Service Attendance by Gender and LGBT Orientation.

Fifty-three percent of ROAH respondents agreed when asked if they attended religious services on a regular basis. Overall, 30% reported attending services at least weekly, and 22% said they attended at least monthly. The remainder consisted of those attending a few times per year (24%) and those attending once per year or less often (24%). Service attendance was significantly related to both gender and sexual orientation in the ROAH sample. Men and women reported more frequent service attendance as compared with transgender older adults with HIV. In terms of sexual orientation, there was little difference in the proportion of each group reporting weekly or monthly service attendance. But LGBT older adults were more likely than heterosexuals to report that they attended once a year or less often, likely reflecting the persistent homophobia found in many religious congregations (see Figure 2).

EFFECTS OF HIV DIAGNOSIS ON RELIGIOUS PARTICIPATION

Religion and spirituality can benefit the lives of older adults living with HIV. It is regrettable that many of these individuals find their HIV diagnosis creates a barrier to accessing these resources. Cotton and colleagues (2006a) found that one in four people with HIV felt estranged from their place of worship, while one-in-ten had changed their place of worship. Much of this alienation can be explained by HIV stigma which is rooted its association with marginalized groups such as gay men (homophobia) or injection-drug users (Kalichman, 1998; Reece, Tanner, Karpiak, & Coffey, 2007). For many an HIV diagnosis engenders a destructive sense of guilt. The person with HIV may perceive the infection as a punishment for past sins, perhaps mediated by a higher power (Jue & Lewis, 2001; Raman & Winer, 2002; see Chapter VI). For people living with HIV, staying involved with religion may require a change of religious identity or affiliation in order to resolve the discord between institutionalized homophobia or HIV-based stigma and their own experience as a person of faith (Miller, 2005a; Seegers, 2007).

ROAH participants were asked whether or not their HIV diagnosis had affected their religious participation; over two-thirds (69%) said that it had not. Of the remainder, one-half (16%) said they attended more frequently, and the other half (15%) reported attending less frequently. Forty-four percent of ROAH respondents had turned to religious congregations for support. These individuals reported that their congregations supported them emotionally and spiritually, and in a few instances, provided instrumental help with transportation, frequently connected with attending services, or bringing meals to the home. For those who did not seek support, the primary reasons were stigma and the fear of rejection and judgment they would encounter if their HIV diagnosis were disclosed or discovered. Despite the subgroup differences in religious affiliation and attendance patterns, these factors were not significantly related to whether or not HIV had affected service attendance or whether they sought support from their religious community.

SPIRITUALITY AND HIV

A diagnosis of HIV may precipitate a development in ones spirituality as existential issues are raised. These include the meaning of life, death and dying, or why the person has become infected and not others (Cotton et al., 2006a; Ironson et al., 2006). A diagnosis of HIV can induce a state of "spiritual distress" (Seegers, 2005) reflecting the depth of disturbance an HIV diagnosis can have on one's belief system. Spiritual distress is often felt as spiritual suffering, doubts about beliefs, withdrawal from others, feelings of being spiritually empty, and perceptions that life is not worth living (Hicks & Lu, 2006). While this distress may be unpleasant, it may in turn foster positive changes in spirituality and religiousness among people living with HIV (Kalichman, 1998).

Table 1. Spirituality Assessment Scale (SAS) Average Scores

	Total		Purpose		Inner		Connected		Transcend	
Group	**M**	**(SD)**	**M**	**(SD)**	**M**	**(SD)**	**M**	**(SD)**	**M**	**(SD)**
Total Sample	135.5	(25.9)	19.8	(4.4)	45.1	(9.0)	43.0	(8.6)	27.7	(6.1)
Race /Ethnicity[a]										
White	132.4	(26.8)	18.6	(5.0)	43.3	(9.8)	43.3	(8.0)	27.2	(6.1)
Black	139.7	(22.6)	20.6	(3.8)	47.1	(7.4)	43.7	(7.8)	28.4	(5.6)
Latino	131.9	(27.6)	19.2	(4.8)	43.3	(9.6)	42.3	(9.2)	27.1	(6.4)

Note. N=900 for SAS Total Scale. Ns=900 to 903 for SAS Subscales (i.e., *Purpose* – Purpose and Meaning in Life; *Inner* – Inner Resources; *Connected* – Unifying Inner-Connectedness; and *Transcend* – Transcendence).

[a] For SAS Total Scale $F (2,812) = 1.94$, $p = .15$, SAS Subscales [Race/Ethnicity: Multivariate] $F (8,804) = 3.16, p < .02$.

[b] Significant Between-subject Effects: *Purpose* $F(2, 810) =3.47, p < .01$; *Inner* $F(2, 810) =3.95, p < .01$

ROAH included The Spirituality Assessment Scale (SAS), which measures four dimensions of spirituality (i.e., *Purpose and Meaning in Life*, *Inner Resources*, *Unifying Interconnectedness* and *Transcendence*; Howden, 1992). The average SAS score among ROAH participants was 135.5 (see Table 1). Average subscale scores on the SAS ranged from 19.8 for *Purpose and Meaning* to 45.1 for *Inner Resources*. There were no significant differences in average SAS total scores by gender, race/ethnicity, or sexual orientation, reflecting the importance of spirituality in this population regardless of background. Analysis of SAS subscale scores revealed a relationship with these measures and race/ethnicity (see Table 1). Overall, Blacks had the highest subscale scores which was most evident for *Purpose and Meaning in Life* and *Inner Resources*.

A COMPARISON OF RELIGION AND SPIRITUALITY IN ROAH

How similar or different is the ROAH sample from other groups of adults concerning religion and spirituality? One study of HIV/AIDS with a younger sample (*M* age = 43 years), predominantly male (86%) and of minority race/ethnicity (55%), found that 23% attended services on a weekly basis (Cotton et al., 2006a), while 30% of ROAH participants attended weekly. The higher proportion of frequent attendees in the ROAH cohort may be related to the greater proportion of women and people of color in this group who are more likely to attend frequently as compared to men or Whites (Clark, 2000; Fitchett et al., 2007).

How do ROAH participants compare to other groups who do not have HIV? One comparable group with a life altering chronic condition is older adults with visual impairment or blindness. This is can be an appropriate comparison group because blindness is also a highly stigmatized condition that has been historically been viewed as "punishment for sin" in both Judeo-Christian and non-Christian traditions (e.g., Oedipus Rex; Brennan & Silverstone, 2000). Secondly, research finds that the burden of disease associated with visual impairment and blindness is similar to that of living with HIV/AIDS because of its life-altering nature and the absence of a cure (see G. C. Brown et al., 2005; M. M. Brown et al., 2005).

One recent study of visual impairment among adults 45 years and older (Brennan, 2004; Brennan & Lee, in press) provides some insight into understanding the interrelationships of HIV and spirituality and religiousness. The visual impairment sample was older than ROAH (i.e., 67 years vs. 56 years on average), and contained a higher proportions of both women (64%) and Whites (64%), and the college-educated (approximately 50%). Both groups were residents of New York City. Despite these differences, levels of attendance between the two groups are remarkably similar. Fifty-two percent of ROAH respondents attended services on at least a monthly basis, while 50% of the visually impaired sample attended services as frequently. However, older adults with vision loss were more likely to attend at least weekly (35%) as compared with 22% of ROAH respondents.

Table 2. Comparison of Spiritual Assessment Scale (SAS) Scores between ROAH participants and Older Adults with Visual Impairment or Blindness

	ROAH		Visually Impaired		t-value
	M	*(SD)*	*M*	*(SD)*	
Total Scale	135.5	(25.9)	134.5	(17.1)	0.51
Purpose & Meaning	19.8	(4.4)	19.0	(3.5)	2.35*
Inner Resources	45.1	(9.0)	44.3	(6.3)	1.17
Inner Connectedness	43.0	(8.6)	44.0	(5.6)	1.53
Transcendence	27.7	(6.1)	27.0	(4.9)	1.48

Note. ROAH; N = 900 to 903. Visually Impaired; N = 188 to 190.
* $p < .05$ independent t-test.

Table 2 shows a comparison of SAS total and subscale scores between ROAH participants and a visually impaired group. Not only were there no significant differences between these two groups in SAS total scale scores or on three of the four subscales, but the scores were almost identical. ROAH respondents did have significantly higher average scores on the SAS *Purpose and Meaning* subscale. This finding reflects other research on spirituality and HIV which finds a heightened quest for meaning in life following an HIV/AIDs diagnosis (Dunphy, 1987; Gehr, 2002; Kalichman, 1998). Overall there is a remarkable similarity between older adults living with HIV and those who are visually impaired or blind regarding religious participation and spirituality. These findings support the contention that the spiritual and religious resources of the older population with HIV should be considered when proposing how to best address the needs of this group.

CONCLUSIONS

Older adults will be the largest group of people living with HIV in the next decade Spirituality has important implications for both physical health and psychological well-being. However, as the ROAH data show, many are estranged from their religious congregations due to the stigma of HIV/AIDS, homosexuality or drug use. AIDS phobia and homophobia have been sanctioned and encouraged by many religious teachings and religious leaders (Miller, 2007; Tibesar, 1986). HIV continues to be perceived as a "gay" disease because of its emergence in that population in the 1980s. Such stigma, whether it results in ostracism or withdrawal from religious participation, can prevent access to important social support and spiritual resources at a time when their needs are greatest.

The majority of older adults in ROAH are persons of color, whose communities have historically embraced religious institutions which often provided a safe haven from a hostile majority culture. ROAH shows that older adults with HIV are resilient, continuing to attend or increasing their attendance at services, and possessing levels of spirituality comparable to other individuals confronting serious, incurable medical conditions. Given the traditional importance of spirituality and religion in the lives of many ROAH respondents, it is not surprising that those who lack these personal resources are also more socially isolated, lonely and depressed (Brennan, Cantor, Shippy, & Karpiak, 2008). But on the positive side, those who are spiritually resilient following their HIV diagnosis are able to maintain these important connections that appear to ameliorate the experience of stigma and protect against mental distress (Brennan, Vance, Shippy, & Karpiak, 2008).

It is not surprising that religion and spirituality have been linked to a number of positive outcomes in other research on people with HIV, including reduced HIV symptoms and lowered stress and distress (Chibnall, Videen, Duckro, & Miller, 2002; Holzemer, Spicer, Wilson, Kemppainen, & Coleman, 1998; Phillips, Mock, Bopp, Dudgeon, & Hand, 2006; Tuck, McCain, & Elswick, 2001). Spirituality appears to provide protection against depression in a range of HIV-positive populations, including males and racial/ethnic minorities (Simoni & Ortiz, 2003; Yi et al., 2006). Spirituality has also been associated with other positive psychosocial outcomes in people with HIV such as health-related quality-of-life, cognitive and social functioning, and emotional well-being (Coleman, 2003; Frame, Uphold, Shehan, & Reid, 2005; McKelroy & Vosvick, 2006).

Some of the more significant findings on spirituality and HIV among older adults are their relationships to risk behaviors and medication adherence. Failure to adhere to HAART can result in a failure to halt the progression of the disease, the development of treatment-resistant strains of the virus, and a higher risk of infecting others (Parsons, Cruise, Davenport, & Jones, 2006; Simoni, Frick, & Huang, 2006). Higher levels of spirituality have been found to be associated with increased adherence to HAART among adults with HIV in a variety of populations (Holstad, Pace, De, & Ura, 2006; Simoni et al.). Greater spirituality is also related to a decrease in HIV-risk behaviors, such as drug use and failure to use condoms (Avants, Marcotte, Arnold, & Margolin, 2003; Simoni, Martone, & Kerwin, 2002). It is important to recognize that not everyone is spiritually inclined and no one should be coerced to participate in religious and spiritual activities (DePalo & Brennan, 2005). However, being sensitive and acknowledging the intrinsic religious and spiritual needs of older adults with HIV in the context of providing services is likely to improve health outcomes and quality of life.

REFERENCES

Avants, S. K., Marcotte, D., Arnold, R., & Margolin, A. (2003). Spiritual beliefs, world assumptions, and HIV risk behavior among heroin and cocaine users. *Psychology of Addictive Behaviors, 17*(2), 159-162.

Brennan, M. (2004). Spirituality and religiousness predict adaptation to vision loss among middle-age and older adults. *International Journal for the Psychology of Religion, 14* (3), 193-214.

Brennan, M., Cantor, M. H., Shippy, R. A., & Karpiak, S. E. (August, 2008). Loneliness and social isolation of older adults living with HIV. Poster session presented at the 17th International AIDS Conference, Mexico City, Mexico.

Brennan, M., & Lee, E. (in press). Untangling the relationships between religiousness, social networks, and the variety and quality of social support among middle-aged and older adults with visual impairment. In A. L. Ai and M. Ardelt (Eds.), *The role of faith in the well-being of older adults: Linking theories with evidence in an interdisciplinary inquiry.* Hauppauge, NY: Nova Science Publishers.

Brennan, M., & Silverstone, B. (2000). Developmental perspectives of aging and vision loss. In B. Silverstone, M. A. Lang, B. Rosenthal, & E. Faye (Eds.), *The Lighthouse handbook on vision impairment and rehabilitation, Vol. I.,* (pp. 409-430). New York: Oxford University Press.

Brennan, M., Vance, D. E., Shippy, R. A., & Karpiak, S. E. (August, 2008). Stigma, spiritual abuse, and resilience among older adults with HIV. Paper presented in the symposium, "Resilience in spiritual communities despite stigma, abuse and restriction" (C. E. Agaibi & R. D. Hetzel, Co-Chairs), American Psychological Association, Boston, MA. August 15, 2008.

Brown, G. C., Brown, M. M., Sharma, S., Stein, J. D., Roth, Z., Campanella, J., & Beauchamp, G. R. (2005). The burden of age-related macular degeneration: A value-based medicine analysis. *Transactions of the American Ophthalmologic Society, 103,* 173-186.

Brown, M. M., Brown, G. C., Stein, J. D., Roth, Z., Campanella, J., & Beauchamp, G. R. (2005). Age-related macular degeneration: Economic burden and value-based medicine analysis. *Canadian Journal of Ophthalmology, 40,* 277-287.

Chibnall, J. T., Videen, S. D., Duckro, P. N., & Miller, D. K. (2002). Psychosocial-spiritual correlates of death distress in patients with life-threatening medical conditions. *Palliative Medicine, 16*(4), 331-8.

Clark, W. (2000). Patterns of religious attendance. *Canadian Social Trends, Statistics Canada — Catalogue No. 11-008,* 23-27.

Coleman, C. L. (2003). Spirituality and sexual orientation: Relationship to mental well-being and functional health status. *Journal of Advanced Nursing, 43*(5), 457-64.

Cotton, S., Tsevat, J., Szaflarski, M., et al. (2006a). Changes in religiousness and spirituality attributed to HIV/AIDS: Are there age and sex differences? *Journal of General Internal Medicine 21,* (Suppl 5), S14-20.

DePalo, R., & Brennan, M. (2005). Spiritual caregiving for older adults: A perspective from clinical practice. In M. Brennan and D. Heiser (Eds.), *Spiritual assessment and intervention with older adults: Current directions and applications*, (pp. 151-160). Binghamton, NY: Haworth Pastoral Press.

Dunphy, R. (1987). Helping persons with AIDS find meaning and hope. *Health Progress, 68*(4), 58-63.

Espinosa, G. (2008). The influence of religion on Latino education, marriage, and social views in the United States. *Marriage & Family Review, 43* (3/4), 205-26.

Fitchett, G., Murphy, P. E., Kravitz, H. M., Everson-Rose, S. A., Krause, N. M., & Powell, L. H. (2007). Racial/ethnic differences in religious involvement in a multi-ethnic cohort of midlife women. *Journal for the Scientific Study of Religion, 46* (1), 119-33.

Frame, M. W., Uphold, C. R., Shehan, C. L., & Ried, K. J. (2005). Effects of spirituality on health-related quality of life in men with HIV/AIDS: Implications for counseling. *Counseling and Values, 50*(1), 5-19.

Gehr, F. C. (2002). Spiritual experiences of HIV-positive gay males: A phenomenological investigation. *Dissertation Abstracts International: Section B: The Sciences and Engineering, 63*(2-B), 1025.

Heinrich, C. R. (2003). Enhancing the perceived health of HIV seropositive men. *Western Journal of Nursing Research, 25*(4), 383-7.

Hicks, D. W., & Lu, F. G. (2006). Religious and spiritual considerations. In F. Fernandez and P. Ruiz (Eds.), *Psychiatric aspects of HIV/AIDS* (pp. 347-354). Philadelphia, PA: Lippincott Williams and Wilkins Publishers.

Holstad, M. K. M., Pace, J. C., De, A. K., & Ura, D. R. (2006). Factors associated with adherence to antiretroviral therapy. *Journal of the Association of Nurses in AIDS Care, 17*(2), 4-15.

Holzemer, W. L., Spicer, J. G., Wilson, H. S., Kemppainen, J. K., & Coleman, C. (1998). Validation of the quality of life scale: living with HIV. *Journal of Advanced Nursing, 28*(3), 622-630.

Howden, J. (1992). *Development and psychometric characteristics of the Spirituality Assessment Scale.* Unpublished doctoral dissertation. Texas Women's University.

Ironson, G., Stuetzle, R., & Fletcher, M. A. (2006). An increase in religiousness/spirituality occurs after HIV diagnosis and predicts slower disease progression over 4 years in people with HIV. *Journal of General Internal Medicine, 21*(Suppl 5), S62-68.

Jue, S., & Lewis, S. Y. (2001). Cultural considerations in HIV ethical decision making: A guide for mental health practitioners. In J. R. Anderson and R. L. Barret (Eds.), *Ethics in HIV-related psychotherapy: Clinical decision making in complex cases* (pp. 61-82). Washington, DC: American Psychological Association.

Kalichman, S. C. (1998). Coping, adjustment, and social support." *Understanding AIDS: Advances in research and treatment* (pp. 257-287). Washington, DC: American Psychological Association.

Kendall, J. (1994). Wellness spirituality in homosexual men with HIV infection. *The Journal of the Association of Nurses in AIDS Care, 5*(4), 28-34.

Lewis, C. E. Jr., & Trulear, H. D. (2008-09). Rethinking the role of African American churches as social service providers. *Black Theology: An International Journal, 6* ,343-66

Lindgren, K. N., & Coursey, R. D. (1995). Spirituality and serious mental illness: A two-part study. *Psychosocial Rehabilitation Journal, 18,* 93-107.

Lorenz, K. A., Hays, R. D., Shapiro, M. F., Cleary, P. D., Asch, S. M., & Wenger, N. S. (2005). Religiousness and spirituality among HIV-infected Americans. *Journal of Palliative Medicine, 8*(4), 774-781.

McKelroy, J. L., & Vosvick, M. (2006). Spirituality and psychological quality of life in HIV+ adults. Paper session presented at the 114th Annual Convention of the American Psychological Association, August 10-13, 2006, New Orleans, LA.

Miller, R. L. (2005a). An appointment with god: AIDS, place, and spirituality. *Journal of Sex Research, 42*(1), 35-45.

Miller, R. L. (2005b). Look what God can do: African American gay men, AIDS and spirituality. *Journal of HIV/AIDS and Social Services, 4*(3), 25-46.

Miller, R. L. (2007). Legacy denied: African American gay men, AIDS, and the black church. *Social Work, 52*(1): 51-61.

Moberg, D. O. (1967). Science and the spiritual nature of man. *Journal of the American Scientific Affiliation, 19,* 12-17.

Pargament, K. I. (1997). *The psychology of religion and coping.* New York: Guilford Press.

Parsons, S. K., Cruise, P. L., Davenport, W. M., & Jones, V. (2006). Religious beliefs, practices and treatment adherence among individuals with HIV in the Southern United States. *AIDS Patient Care and STDs, 20*(2), 97-111.

Phillips, K. D., Mock, K. S., Bopp, C. M., Dudgeon, W. A., & Hand, G. A. (2006). Spiritual well-being, sleep disturbance, and mental and physical health status in HIV-infected individuals. *Issues in Mental Health Nursing, 27*(2), 125-139.

Raman, L., & Winer, G. A. (2002). Children's and adults' understanding of illness: Evidence in support of a coexistence model. *Genetic, Social, and General Psychology Monographs, 128*(4), 325-55.

Reece, M., Tanner, A. E., Karpiak, S. E., & Coffey, K. (2007). The impact of HIV-related stigma on HIV care and prevention providers. *Journal of HIV/AIDS and Social Services, 6*(3), 55-73.

Seegers, D. L. (2005). Spiritual and religious experiences of gay men with HIV illness. *Dissertation Abstracts International: Section B: The Sciences and Engineering 66,* (6-B): 3063.

Seegers, D. L. (2007). Spiritual and religious experiences of gay men with HIV illness. *The Journal of the Association of Nurses in AIDS Care, 18*(3), 5-12.

Siegel, K., & Schrimshaw, E. W. (2002). The perceived benefits of religious and spiritual coping among older adults living with HIV. *Journal for the Scientific Study of Religion, 41*(1), 91-102.

Simoni, J. M., Frick, P. A., & Huang, B. (2006). A longitudinal evaluation of a social support model of medication adherence among HIV-positive men and women on antiretroviral therapy. *Health Psychology, 25*(1), 74-81.

Simoni, J. M., Martone, M. G., & Kerwin, J. F. (2002). Spirituality and psychological adaptation among women with HIV/AIDS: Implications for counseling. *Journal of Counseling Psychology, 49*(2), 139-47.

Simoni, J. M., & Ortiz, M. Z. (2003). Mediational models of spirituality and depressive symptomatology among HIV-positive Puerto Rican women. *Cultural Diversity and Ethnic Minority Psychology, 9*(1), 3-15.

Tibesar, L. J. (1986). AIDS: Responding to the crisis. Pastoral care: Helping patients on an inward journey. *Health Progress, 67*(4), 41-7.

Tuck, I., McCain, N. L., & Elswick, R. K. Jr. (2001). Spirituality and psychosocial factors in persons living with HIV. *Journal of Advanced Nursing, 33*(6), 776-83.

Yi, M. S., Mrus, J. M., Wade, T. J., et al. 2006. Religion, spirituality, and depressive symptoms in patients with HIV/AIDS. *Journal of General Internal Medicine, 21*(Suppl 5), S21-S27.

In: Older Adults with HIV
Editors: M. Brennan, S.E. Karpiak et al.
ISBN 978-1-60876-054-1
© 2009 Nova Science Publishers, Inc.

Chapter 11

AGING WITH HIV: IMPLICATIONS AND FUTURE DIRECTIONS

Stephen E. Karpiak and Mark Brennan

This volume has documented the evolution of people living with HIV; each year there are more and more people growing older with this condition. In New York City the number of older adults over age 50 with HIV has been increasing at the rate of 2% annually (New York City Department of Health and Mental Hygiene, 2001; 2008). Using a conservative calculation, we have estimated that by 2015, over 50% of those living with HIV in New York City will be 50 and older (Brennan, 2008). Further, the number of people living with HIV 65 and older has increased more than tenfold in the last decade (Stoff et al., 2004). This graying of the HIV epidemic is all too often overlooked. But change is coming and it will require that policy makers, program planners, service providers, and researchers develop new paradigms to address this changing landscape.

How then can our communities provide optimal care for these older adults who have been given the hope of a long life due to the effectiveness of anti-retroviral therapies? Health care providers have focused on optimizing the medical treatment regimens needed to control HIV infection and its consequences. The effectiveness of this approach is measured in the dramatic reduction in mortality rates, the rise in CD4 immune cells and the drop in viral loads for those living with HIV. However, it is imperative that we broaden this focus to beyond the medical to address the myriad challenges faced by people growing older with HIV.

THE CHALLENGE OF MANAGING MULTIPLE CHRONIC ILLNESSES

HIV is taking its place as one of many chronic illnesses, but the evolution of people living with HIV into aging, long-term survivors demands a revolution in HIV care. In addition to the comorbidities associated with HIV and its treatments, the comorbidities associated with aging are occurring in this population at an unusually young age. ROAH finds that these relatively young respondents (average age = 56) report 3 times as many comorbid conditions as adults 70 and older (Chapter II). It is not clear why this is happening, but this pattern is being seen and reported in many clinical settings. As observed in Chapter II, *"...these comorbidities represent a mixture of the effects of the virus itself. While anti-retrovirals protect the immune system from collapse due to HIV infection, the virus is likely exerting effects on other organ systems and tissue metabolic activities. These HIV effects may be contributing to the seemingly early onset and severity of age associated illnesses."*

The challenge of managing the older adult with HIV will be substantial. The present medical care system focuses on HIV infection and is not attuned to the effective management of multiple comorbid conditions. Often comorbidities are each treated by a different medical care provider as if they occur in isolation when a holistic approach is needed. Treatment that is ideal for a specific illness is not necessarily good for the person as a whole since the management of one disease can complicate and even worsen other conditions. The Ryan White Care Act, which started in 1990, is the largest federal program designed specifically for people with HIV/AIDS. A minimum of 75% of these funds are used for "core medical services" which translates into the cost and care associated with HAART (Kaiser Family Foundation, 2009). As a result, Ryan White funding streams are largely used to support clinical services for HIV. There are frequent reassessments and changes in standards of care for the management of HIV. However, other conditions that are treated in the context of HIV care are often considered secondary with the primary focus, logically, placed on the management of HIV. For these other illnesses, the standards of care are not as rigorously assessed to determine if they indeed insure the best level of care possible as evidenced by positive outcomes. One example of this is the high levels of depression seen in the HIV population which is the result of poor management of this comorbidity. Thus, standards-of-care may need to be reexamined that are not producing expected outcomes for people living with HIV (Chapter III).

RECOMMENDATIONS

- As older people live longer with HIV, reexamine and modify standards-of-care for HIV to include routine assessments for the myriad comorbid illnesses that are common among aging adults. These assessments must be implemented at an earlier age due to the accelerated aging observed in this population.
- Provide funding for the development of geriatric curricula at medical schools and universities that train medical students, other medical providers, and aging specialists about the particular needs of the over-50 HIV-positive population.
- Assess the problematic interactions that are likely between antiretrovirals and those drugs use to treat the common comorbidities associated with aging.
- Ensure that older men and women are included as identifiable groups at every stage of the HIV medical and pharmacological research process.
- Increase funding from government agencies and private foundations for basic research into the particular physical and mental health needs and experiences of older adults with HIV. Such research should include:
  - Interactions between HIV and the common diseases and chronic conditions of older adults.

- Targeted research aimed at treating depression and other mental health problems simultaneously among older adults with HIV, including substance use and sexual risk-taking. The co-occurrence model as recently funded by the New York State Health Foundation is an example of a new, needed and data-driven approach (see Chapter IV).
- Evaluation of existing medical, health and social services use and their effectiveness for older adults with HIV.

HIV AND AGING:
PSYCHOSOCIAL FACTORS CANNOT BE MARGINALIZED

The medical model is not sufficient to optimally manage people living with HIV as they age into their 50s and beyond. As the person with HIV ages, it is incumbent upon medical providers and caregivers alike to understand the best care practices for older adults. Psychosocial factors must be considered when treatment decisions are made regarding HIV or other illnesses. For example, the high prevalence of depression and other mental health problems are critical issues that must be considered and resolved because they interfere with adherence to medication and rehabilitation regimens (see Chapter III).

More than 70% of ROAH respondents live alone and often have little support from family or friends. Adherence to the complex medical regimens of HAART is facilitated by having a spouse, partner or nearby friend or neighbor who can provide informal support and caregiving, which is essential for successful aging (e.g., Wrubel, Stubmo, & Johnson, 2008). The fragile social networks found in ROAH as evidenced by the lack of functional network members (Chapter VII), as well as the high levels of social isolation and loneliness reported (Chapter VIII), do not constitute an optimal environment for managing complex, multiple illnesses. This situation is exacerbated by the history of substance use and the concomitant reliance on recovery programs. These are significant factors that shape the lives of many older adults with HIV.

In addition, the loneliness and social isolation seen in ROAH suggest that many in the population are in need of greater opportunities to socialize and connect with others. Socialization is a key factor as a predictor of successful aging. The ROAH group as a whole is not very engaged socially. Stigma may render them afraid to access social support services, like senior centers, which provide human contact and specific types of support. But the high levels of spirituality and frequent attendance at religious services among ROAH respondents (see Chapter X), as well considerable resilience as evidenced by their psychological well-being (Chapter IX) suggest that this group has the resources to overcome these limitations if presented with the opportunities to do so.

Considering the limited funding available for caring for people with HIV, how can our society best address the confluence of medical and psychosocial needs that this population will experience as it ages? How do we draw on the strengths that already exist in these older adults and the communities where they live? Existing resources must be accessed and integrated into the lives of older adults with HIV. AIDS service organizations (ASOs) and other community-based organizations (CBOs) are not going to be able to retool themselves to address the massive demands of the aging process. Older adults living with HIV must feel safe to engage the health and social support systems that nearly every other aging adult in the U.S. can access. Mainstreaming is needed, and through mainstreaming stigma will be reduced. Older adults with HIV must empower and educate themselves regarding aging issues and be prepared to engage their health providers with their needs and concerns. There is a need to create relationships between the array of aging support services and the ASO/CBO networks.

RECOMMENDATIONS

- The Older Americans Act (OAA) should be amended explicitly to include services, outreach, training, and research on issues of concern to older HIV-positive older adults and to prohibit discrimination by providers who take these funds on the basis of HIV status and sexual orientation. These changes should be accompanied by new funding to pay for the services, so that funds are not simply redirected away from other at-risk groups.
- ASO and CBO staff should receive ongoing training on aging and the particular needs of older adults with HIV and such training should be funded through the OAA, Ryan White Care Act, or other federal, state or local programs.
- ASO staff should work with their Area Agencies on Aging (AAAs) to assess the needs of older adults with HIV, evaluate whether those needs are being met by community-based services and influence their area plans to ensure that older adults with HIV have the services they need and deserve.
- Training and education on the needs of older adults with HIV can decrease stigma and create a safe environment in which these older adults can partake fully of services offered to other elders. HIV-positive adults (i.e., peer educators) should be included as both trainers and advisors. This training should target senior center staff, homecare workers, social workers, and other ageing service providers. Such training should increase the availability of programs and services that are sensitive to this aging HIV population and responsive to its needs.
- CBOs and ASOs should apply for demonstration funding to provide training on HIV to those who provide services to older adults with this condition under OAA, Part F, which provides for state and local innovation and programs of national significance.
- Develop collaborations between senior centers and CBOs/ASOs already providing services to older adults with HIV. Such collaboration should involve better outreach coordination by ASOs/CBOs and aging service providers to HIV-positive older adults to join in the socialization activities and other programs in senior centers.
- Maintain the inclusive language in Part E of the National Family Caregiver Support Program that defines family caregiver as "an adult family member, or another individual, who is an informal provider of in-home and community care to an older individual."
- Demonstration projects should be undertaken to strengthen the role of family and friends in the informal support network in providing care for older people with HIV, including the specific needs of these individuals and how best they can provide support.

- Increase knowledge, through research, about how stigma continues to prevent people from disclosing their HIV status to others, thus limiting the availability and adequacy of support they receive from family, friends and others.

EXPANDING HIV PREVENTION EFFORTS TO INCLUDE OLDER ADULTS

Rarely do HIV prevention programs include older adults with most focusing on adolescents and young adults. The need to develop age-relevant prevention materials and interventions is needed beyond posting information on web sites. Adults 50 and older do not fall into the category of a high-risk group because most HIV infections occur between the ages of 25 and 49. However, recent data indicate that 15% of all new HIV infections occur among those 50 and older (Center for Disease Control and Prevention [CDC], 2008), and new epidemiological data suggests that the proportion is increasing. It is also likely that there is an underreporting of HIV cases in the 50 and older population given that HIV testing is not seen as important for this group. As the number of older adults living with HIV increases, the likelihood of a noninfected person in this cohort encountering a HIV-positive age-peer increases. As we report in ROAH (Chapter V) and as Cooperman and colleagues (2007) have documented, a sizeable minority HIV-positive older adults continue to engage in unsafe sex behavior.

There is a failure of the HIV prevention network and medical providers to include older adults in programs and to sensitize older adults to the fact that they too are at-risk (Akers, Bernstein, Doyle, & Corbie-Smith, 2008). As a result, many older adults fail to get tested while they still have an early-stage HIV infection. This is starkly illustrated by recent epidemiological data (CDC, 2007). Among adults 50 and older who received a diagnosis of HIV infection, 51% also received an AIDS diagnosis within 12 months as compared with 33% of those in the younger age groups. Most new infections occur because the person passing the virus to another does not know they have HIV. What is particularly disturbing about this high incidence of AIDS diagnoses in the older population is the fact that when a person is HIV-positive and has progressed to the advanced stage of the illness (i.e., AIDS), they are highly infectious due to high levels of the virus in their bodies. A person with HIV who is on HAART typically has viral levels that are low and often undetectable.

The New York City Council is the only government entity to-date that has recognized the need to bring HIV information and prevention efforts to older adults in their communities. Starting in 2007, the New York City Council has funded three one-year initiatives to address this need. ACRIA (AIDS Community Research Initiative of America) has been the lead agency creating collaborations among those who provide services to older adults and other AIDS service organizations in New York.[1] While this issue is beginning to be addressed across the country (Altschuler, Katz, & Tynan, 2004; Orel, Wright, & Wagner, 2004), much more needs to be done to eliminate HIV infections in the 50 and older age group.

---

[1] For more information on ACRIA's HIV Health Literacy training programs and materials on HIV prevention for older adults, please visit www.acria.org .

RECOMMENDATIONS

- Tailor and target HIV effective prevention messages to older adults.
- Develop prevention interventions that are age and group appropriate.
- Increase testing for HIV in the over 50 population.
- Sensitize medical care providers to the need to discuss risk behaviors with all clients, including, not excluding, older adults.
- Increase knowledge through research about how stigma continues to discourage HIV-testing and prevents older adults from disclosing their serostatus to others.

CONCLUSION

ROAH underlines a destructive issue that remains within our society; the intense loneliness, social isolation and depression that can largely be traced to the power of HIV stigma (Chapter VI). At its root, this stigma is driven by homophobia which is particularly intense within communities of color. HIV stigma is rooted in misinformation, myths, and fear. Stigma affects health, and is a factor which fuels HIV infection rates by discouraging HIV testing and encouraging secrecy and shame. Stigma is the factor which will essentially prevent these older adults with HIV from accessing the social care they will need from family, friends, neighbors and their community. This is not only an economic or medical issue, but a human issue that is given cursory lip service by too many government and community leaders and the social institutions they represent, including the vast network of faith-based communities. All must share in the responsibility for the neglect of their members most in need of care due to HIV regardless of age.

Massive efforts have given life and hope where none existed a decade ago. Prolonged life has been given, but for too many it is a life riddled with loneliness, isolation, fear, rejection and guilt. There is a price to be paid for this extreme prejudice, this ease with which one judges another person who has a health issue. Without the support from their family, friends, and communities, the caregiving which these older adults with HIV will need will place further demands on a healthcare system that is already inadequate and under duress. The successes and failures of the management of the HIV epidemic and the treatment of HIV is a microcosm of the challenges which the U.S. faces in its present attempt to restructure the health care system. Part of this restructuring will include taking responsibility for oneself and for all the members of our communities. How we will respond to this challenge will define who we are.

REFERENCES

Akers, A. Y., Bernstein, L., Doyle, J., & Corbie-Smith, G. (2008). Older women and HIV testing: Examining the relationship between HIV testing history, age, and lifetime HIV risk behaviors. *Sexually Transmitted Diseases, 35*(4), 420-423.

Altschuler, J. Katz, A. D., & Tynan, M. (2004). Developing and implementing and HIV/AIDS educational curriculum for older adults. *The Gerontologist, 44*(1), 121-6.

Brennan, M. (2008). Keynote address. Colloquium, *A graying epidemic: HIV/AIDS and older adults,* presented by the School of Social Work and Center on Aging, University of Maine, September 26, 2008.

CDC [Center for Disease Control and Prevention]. (2007). *HIV/AIDS Surveillance Report, 19.* Retrieved December 2, 2008 from the World Wide Web: http://cdc.gov/hiv/topics/surveillance/resources/reports/2007report/pdf/2007SurveillanceReport.pdf

CDC [Center for Disease Control and Prevention]. (2008). HIV/AIDS among persons 50 and older. Retrieved May 19, 2008 from the World Wide Web: http://www.cdc.gov/hiv/topics/over50/resources/factsheets/pdf/over50.pdf

Cooperman, N. A., Arnsten, J. H., & Klein, R. S. (2007). Current sexual activity and risky sexual behavior in older men with or at risk for HIV infection. *AIDS Education and Prevention, 19*(4), 321-333.

Kaiser Family Foundation (2009). HIV/AIDS policy fact sheet: The Ryan White Program. Retrieved March 11, 2009 from the World Wide Web: http://www.kff.org/hivaids/upload/7582_05.pdf

New York City Department of Health and Mental Hygiene (2001). New York City HIV/AIDS annual surveillance statistics 2001. Retrieved November 30, 2008 from the World Wide Web: http://www.nyc.gov/html/doh/downloads/pdf/ah/surveillance 2001_tables_all.pdf

New York City Department of Health and Mental Hygiene (2008). HIV epidemiology and field services semiannual report. Retrieved November 30, 2008 from the World Wide Web: http://www.nyc.gov/html/doh/downloads/pdf/dires/dires-2008-report-semi1.pdf

Stoff, D. M., Khalsa, J. H., Monjan, A., Portegies, P. (2004). Introduction: HIV/AIDS and Aging. *AIDS, 18* (Suppl 1) S1-2.

Wrubel, J., Stubmo, S., & Johnson, M. O. (2008). Antiretroviral medication support practices among partners of men who have sex with men: A qualitative study. *AIDS Patient Care and STDs, 22*(11), 851-8.

ABOUT THE AUTHORS

Allison J. Applebaum, MA, is a doctoral candidate in the Department of Clinical Psychology at Boston University, and is completing her internship in clinical psychology at New York Presbyterian Hospital/Weill-Cornell Medical Center. For the past two years, she has worked as a study interventionist and research assistant in the Behavioral Medicine Service at Massachusetts General Hospital. Ms. Applebaum's clinical and research interests include the neuropsychological sequelae and psychosocial aspects of HIV infection, behavioral medicine, mood and anxiety disorders, and factors that impact the therapeutic alliance.

Mark Brennan, PhD, is a Senior Research Scientist at ACRIA. Dr. Brennan joined ACRIA in 2007 to conduct behavioral research on psychosocial issues affecting persons living with HIV, with a special focus on older adults. Prior to receiving his doctoral degree in Applied Developmental Psychology from Fordham University in 1995, he was a Brookdale Fellow under the mentorship of Professor Marjorie Cantor and served as Co-Principal Investigator on *Growing Older in New York City in the 1990s*. After working at the New York City Department for the Aging, he joined Lighthouse International in 1996 to study coping and adjustment to age-related visual impairment, dual sensory loss of vision and hearing, and the roles of religion and spirituality in adaptation to chronic illness. During his tenure at the Lighthouse, Dr. Brennan served as a Principal Investigator on a study of caregiving among older LGBT adults. Since coming to ACRIA, Dr. Brennan's work has focused on depression, social supports, and spirituality among older adults with HIV, as well as dissemination of the ROAH study. He is currently President-Elect of the State Society on Aging of New York, a Fellow of the Gerontological Society of America (GSA), and Board Member of the New York Association on HIV over Fifty (NYAHOF). He is the Principal Convener for GSA's Religion, Spirituality and Aging formal interest group and the Book Review Editor for the *Journal or Religion, Spirituality and Aging*. Dr. Brennan has been recognized for his research and work in the field of aging by the Hunter-Brookdale Center on Aging, Pride Senior Network, and the New York State Office for the Aging. He has authored over 50 peer-reviewed articles, chapters and books.

Marjorie H. Cantor, MA, is Professor Emerita and Brookdale Distinguished Scholar of Fordham University's Graduate of Social Service. Professor Cantor is a nationally and internationally recognized leader in the field of aging. A past President of the Gerontological Society of America, she was the first Director of Research for the New York City Department for the Aging. Professor Cantor most recently served as a Principal Investigator on the major cross-ethnic study, *Growing Older in New York City in the 1990's,* and has been the Principal Investigator of over nine other large scale studies during her three decades in the field of aging. She is the recipient of numerous awards including the Kent Award (Gerontological Society of America), the Walter M. Beattie, Jr. Award for Distinguished Service in Aging (State Society on Aging of New York), and is a member of the Hunter College Hall of Fame. While at Fordham, Professor Cantor served as the Associate Director of the Third Age Center and Director of the Brookdale Research Center and Doctoral Training Program. She has served as a consultant to numerous Federal, State and local agencies and boards; was a Senior Fellow of the Brookdale Foundation; and was a participant in White House Conferences on Aging (1980 and 1995) and an Invited Participant at the International Forum on Aging hosted by the Chinese Government in Beijing. Her areas of research expertise include elderly in the urban setting, the effect of ethnicity and culture on elderly lifestyles, and the role of family and other informal supports in providing care for older people. She is the author of over 70 articles, books, chapters and papers presented here and abroad.

Sarit A. Golub, PhD, MPH, is an Associate Professor in the Department of Psychology at Hunter College of the City University of New York and Co-Director of the Center for HIV/AIDS Educational Studies and Training. She is also a member of the doctoral faculty in the Neuropsychology and Social-Personality subprograms at the CUNY Graduate Center. Dr. Golub's research interests include the social-cognitive factors that impact clinical, psychological, and behavioral outcomes among individuals living with HIV and those at-risk for future infection.

Julia C. Tomassilli, MPhil, is a doctoral student in the Social/Personality Psychology program at the Graduate Center of the City University of New York and a Senior Research Associate at the Center for HIV/AIDS Educational Studies and Training. Ms. Tomassilli's research interests focus on sexuality and stigma. She has examined the stigmatization of bisexuality and non-normative ("kinky") sexual behaviors and is currently working on her dissertation examining the impact of HIV stigma on the sexual well-being of HIV-positive individuals.

Christian Grov, PhD, MPH, is an Assistant Professor in the Department of Health and Nutrition Sciences at Brooklyn College of the City University of New York. He is also a Faculty Affiliate member of the research team at the Center for HIV/AIDS Educational Studies and Training. Prior to joining Brooklyn College, Dr. Grov received postdoctoral training via the National Development and Research Institutes (NDRI) funded by the National Institute on Drug Abuse. His research centers on the sexual health of gay and bisexual men. In this capacity, his work has explored substance use and the role of the Internet in revolutionizing gay and bisexual men's sexual networks. Dr. Grov has been working in HIV prevention and education since 1999.

Richard J. Havlik, MD, MPH has been a consultant to ACRIA since his retirement from the National Institute on Aging (NIA), part of the National Institutes of Health, Bethesda, Maryland. From 1990 to 2004, Dr. Havlik was Associate Director for Epidemiology, Demography, and Biometry and subsequently Chief of the Laboratory of Epidemiology, Demography, and Biometry in the Intramural Research Program at NIA. He directed a comprehensive program of research into the determinants and correlates of aging and age-associated diseases. His own research has covered a wide range of topics, including cardiovascular disease, cancer, cognitive functioning, dementia and genetic epidemiology. Since 1968, he also held various positions at the National Heart, Lung, and Blood Institute and the National Center for Health Statistics. He is the author of about 100 peer-reviewed publications as well as other chapters, articles, and letters. Dr. Havlik has developed a current interest in the comorbidities associated with aging in HIV patients over 50 years of age.

Stephen Karpiak, PhD has a distinguished career as a research scientist. After obtaining his PhD in 1972, he joined the faculty of Columbia University Medical School with an appointment in Neurology and Psychiatry. At Columbia for over two decades he conducted cutting edge NIH and NSF funded research on the immunological bases of seizures and behavioral disorders. His work showed that antibodies were capable of entering the brain and causing epileptic activity as well as significant behavioral alterations. In 1976 he published a seminal work in *Science* in the field of neuroimmunology. In his last decade at Columbia he achieved international recognition as a researcher by demonstrating that the brain could adapt and repair after injury. His research contributed to changing the widely held belief that in the CNS there was only limited capacity to recover after injury. This work has been part of the rationale for the development of treatments and therapies for the management of peripheral neuropathies, stroke and spinal injury. He has given over 300 invited lectures nationally and internationally and has been a scientific adviser for the United Nations WHO as well as serving on NIH peer review committees. He has published over 100 peer-reviewed articles.

After retiring from Columbia in 1993, Karpiak did his first HIV/AIDS community work in Phoenix. He was a Program Director at *AIDS Project Arizona*, directed its buyers club, and founded the *Arizona AIDS Project Wellness Center*. He later was the Executive Director for *A Place Called Home,* which provided congregate group housing for the homeless with HIV/AIDS using HUD/HOPWA funding. He returned to New York City to become Executive Director for *Pride Senior Network* and for the last seven years has been the Associate Director for Research at the AIDS Community Research Initiative of America (ACRIA). With ACRIA's support he initiated seminal studies on HIV and the aging population. His work has been featured in the media including the New York Times, BBC, CBS, NPR and CNN. Recently he has guided the initiation of a ROAH-London (UK) research effort.

R. Andrew Shippy, MA has conducted gerontological research since 1997. His primary research interests include social support, psychological well-being, caregiving, and personal development in middle age and older adulthood. He has studied the effects of chronic illness and stigma among many vulnerable populations. His work with Dr. Caryn Goodman at Lighthouse International examined the impact of vision impairment on the marital relationship and the mental health of disabled elders and their nondisabled spouses, and his research with Dr. Mark Brennan examined the roles of spirituality and religiousness in coping with vision impairment and personal development among middle-aged and older adults. In 2000, he worked with Professor Cantor and Dr. Brennan on the first large-scale study of the caregiving experiences and needs of LGBT seniors in New York City. His most recent position was as an Associate Research Scientist at ACRIA, where he conducted behavioral research focusing on the growing population of older adults living with HIV. This research examined the impact of personal and social support resources on the quality of life aging adults living with HIV. He has published several articles and presented his research at major national and international scientific and advocacy conferences.

APPENDIX: ROAH METHODOLOGY

SPECIFIC AIMS

The primary goal of this research was to establish empirically valid normative data describing this population and to allow for the analyses of subgroups within the larger population. For example, comparisons of gender, race/ethnicity and sexual orientation can identify potential disparities among these older adults, which will need to be addressed by healthcare providers and policy makers. New York City's HIV population, the largest and most diverse in the United States, is a gauge for changes in the HIV epidemic nationwide. This cohort of aging New Yorkers will be a benchmark against which other studies of aging adults with HIV will be compared. Pending future funding, this cohort will become the baseline data sample of a longitudinal cohort study of older adults with HIV. Before the ROAH study was undertaken, no other group representing the current demographic profile of older adults with HIV existed. Existing cohorts have limited utility because they contain highly selective groups of older adults (e.g., veterans, gay men).

PROJECT SITE

ACRIA is a well-established community-based research organization that has completed over 80 clinical and behavioral studies on HIV, its related diseases, and side effects associated with antiviral medications. ACRIA's research program has existed since 1991, with proven procedures in place to monitor and evaluate progress of individual protocols. These procedures concern multiple aspects of a research project, from timeliness and accuracy with regard to completing all study phases to compliance with HIPAA standards and other practices to protect study participants. The agency has consistently been among the most successful enrollment sites for national multicenter trials of new HIV medications, and has always been in full compliance with FDA regulatory requirements for trials of experimental therapies utilizing human subjects. In fact, a hallmark of ACRIA's work has been a strong focus on ensuring that all populations impacted by HIV have an opportunity to participate in our studies, including vulnerable populations traditionally underserved by HIV research, most prominently ethnic minorities and women.

ACRIA has one of the most extensive networks of partnerships with other community-based organizations and AIDS service organizations of any not-for-profit organization in New York City. This network was used extensively in the recruitment of study participants for the proposed protocol. The agency maintains a database of over 1500 people living with HIV who are interested in receiving information about clinical and behavioral studies at ACRIA. These individuals received IRB-approved recruitment materials for this study.

SAMPLE SELECTION AND RECRUITMENT

As of March 31, 2005, the last date for which data are available, there were approximately 95,707 known cases of HIV in New York City. Of this number, 28,433 (30%) were over age 50. Study participants ($N = 1,000$) were selected from this population. The ROAH study team utilized ACRIA's existing relationships with organizations in New York City to recruit individuals for the study. Recruitment occurred through on-site trainings, presentations and staff visits, as well as mail, telephone and email contacts.

ELIGIBILITY CRITERIA

- confirmed HIV diagnosis.
- age 50 years or older.
- reside in or receive HIV-related healthcare in New York City.
- sufficiently fluent in English to complete the measures.
- community-dwelling (non-institutionalized).
- have no significant cognitive impairment that would preclude completing the study instrument.

INSTRUMENT

The ROAH Program utilized a quantitative, self-administered questionnaire designed by the study investigators, composed of several standardized research measures in addition to items drawn from the investigators' previous work. The instrument was designed to collect detailed information from five general conceptual areas (e.g., physical health, mental health, social support, formal care utilization, and HIV-related stigma and disclosure of HIV serostatus). The instrument has been constructed to yield empirically valid data that can be compared to population norms as well as other studies of HIV-positive individuals. These comparisons will provide a wealth of information about a group of older adults that has been heretofore invisible.

ROAH SURVEY INSTRUMENT MODULES

Module 1: Demographic Profile
- Sociodemographic/background characteristics of individuals.

Module 2: Health Status
- Detailed HIV history including CD4, viral load, when diagnosed, HAART use, etc.
- Past and current substance use, recovery, etc.
- Selected scales from the MOS-HIV will also be used for this module.
- The module contains the 20-item CES-D.

Module 3: Sexual Behaviors
- Sexual behavior checklist includes sexual activities, number of partners, safer sex practices, serostatus of partners, etc.

Module 4: Social Networks
- Perceived network size, functional network size, support satisfaction and support need.
- Independent measures of availability and adequacy of instrumental and emotional support.

Module 5: Stigma
- The Berger HIV Stigma Scale included in this module.
- Level of disclosure, reasons for not disclosing, and level of stigma experienced during interactions with six (biological family, friends, co-workers, social organizations, place of worship, and healthcare providers) groups of people.
- Reasons for nondisclosure

Module 6: Psychological Resources
- Psychological well-being - The absence of physical or mental symptomatology does not imply optimal health. Ryff's scales of psychological well-being encompass six domains (self-acceptance, positive relations with others, autonomy, environmental mastery, purpose in life, and personal growth) that measure positive aspects of well-being.
- Spirituality – Howden Spirituality Assessment Scale is a 28 item instrument with four subscales: 1) Purpose and Meaning in Life, 2) Inner Resources, 3) Unifying Interconnectedness, 4) Transcendence.

MEASURES

- *Demographic profile.* Single items assessed participants' age, race/ethnicity, sex, education, health status, living arrangement, employment status, religious affiliation and participation, sexual orientation, income adequacy, history of incarceration, health coverage, and life satisfaction.
- *HIV status.* Single items assessed date of HIV diagnosis, receipt of an AIDS diagnosis, prior history of HIV testing, CD4 count, HIV infection risk factors, use of

HAART and complementary and alternative medicine use, and type of healthcare provider.

- *Depression.* Depressive symptomatology was measured by the Center for Epidemiologic Studies Depression Scale (CES-D; Radloff, 1977). The CES-D is a 20-item self-report scale designed to assess depressive symptomatology in the general population. The CES-D includes few somatic indicators, thus reducing the likelihood of elevated depression scores due to the physical symptoms common among people living with HIV. Responses are summed to obtain a total symptom score with a range of 0 to 60; higher scores indicate greater depressive symptomatology. Scores below 16 suggest that a person is not depressed. Scores between 16 and 22 indicate moderate levels of depression that would likely correspond with a clinical depression diagnosis, while scores of 23 and above indicate severe levels of depression. This measure has demonstrated high internal consistency (Cronbach's αs = .85 to .90) across diverse community and clinical samples (Radloff, 1977; Ryff & Essex, 1992). In the ROAH sample, the inter-item reliability was also high (i.e., α = .87).

- *Informal support networks.* Detailed information regarding network size and composition, as well as frequency of contact and level of affiliation with network members was collected with an assessment used in previous studies of social networks (Cantor & Brennan, 1993; Cantor, Brennan, & Shippy, 2004; Shippy & Karpiak, 2005a; 2005b). Five groups (e.g., parents, children, siblings, other relatives, and friends), or network elements, that typically comprise informal networks were assessed. Participants indicate if they have any living members of a network element. Three additional items assess frequency of contact with the element (e.g., in-person visits, and telephone conversations) using a five-level Likert-type scale (daily, weekly, monthly, several times a year, once a year or less). A final item assesses the level of closeness within for each network element (e.g., very close, somewhat close, not too close, not close at all). Assessments of contact frequency are necessary to calculate the functional status of each network element, based on criteria established by Cantor (Cantor, 1979). These criteria define the minimum level of contact as either monthly in-person visits or weekly telephone conversations.

- *Support availability and adequacy.* Four items assessed availability and adequacy of informal network support used in previous large-scale studies of New York City's older adults (e.g., Cantor & Brennan, 1993; Cantor et al., 2004). Two identical items provided separate ratings of emotional and instrumental support availability, "Do you have someone you can count on to help you with [type of support]?" Respondents indicated availability on a four-level scale (e.g., most of the time, some of the time, occasionally, or not at all). Adequacy of support was assessed similarly to yield independent ratings for emotional and instrumental support needs. Participants responded to the item, "In the past year, how much more help or assistance with [type of support] did you need," by indicating one of four choices (e.g., needed a lot more, needed some more, needed a little more, or I got all the help I needed).

- *Types and Frequency of Assistance from Family and Friends.* Participants indicated the frequency and types of assistance provided by family members and friends (e.g., two sets of eight positive and three negative types of support that were provided by family and friends in the past month). Each of these responses was scored on a six-point Likert-type scale anchored with 'everyday' and 'not at all'. Responses were summed for each section separately to create a frequency of help provided by family members and friends. These items were adapted from previous studies of older New Yorkers (e.g., Cantor & Brennan, 1993; Cantor et al., 2004).

- *Loneliness.* The UCLA Loneliness Scale (Russell, 1996) is a 20-item measure with high internal consistency (coefficient α = .89 to .94) and acceptable test-retest reliability after one year (r = .73). There are 11 negatively worded items and nine positively worded items in the third version of the scale. Participants responded to items with a four level scale (never, rarely, sometimes, always). The nine positively worded items are reverse coded and scores from all 20 items are summed. Scores range from 20 to 80, and higher scores indicate greater degrees of loneliness. Cronbach's alpha for this measure in the ROAH sample was .90, indicating a high degree of internal consistency.

- *Substance Use.* A substance use checklist assessed both past and current use of 15 different substances (e.g., tobacco, alcohol, cocaine, heroin, etc.). In addition, respondents indicated if, during the past 90 days, they engaged in sexual activities while under the influence of each of these substances.

- *Sexual Behaviors.* Participants answered a series of gender-specific questions regarding their sexual behaviors in the past 90 days. The questions were designed to determine if respondents are involved in seroconcordant relationships or if they engage in sexual activities with HIV-negative partners and individuals who do not disclose their HIV status. In addition, participants reported the number of times they engaged in several behaviors with and without barrier protection (e.g., condoms or dental dams).

- *Health-related quality of life.* Selected subscales (e.g., energy/fatigue, cognitive function, pain, physical function) from the MOS-HIV (Wu et al., 1991) was used to assess health-related quality of life (HRQoL). These subscales were chosen because they assess unique domains not assessed by other measures in the instrument.

- *Psychological well-being.* Ryff's (1989) theoretically-derived scales were used to assess psychological well-being. Each of the six 9-item scales (e.g., Autonomy, Environmental Mastery, Personal Growth, Positive Relations With Others, Purpose in Life, and Self-Acceptance) utilize a 6-point scale ranging from 'strongly agree' to 'strongly disagree' to assess well-being, with scores ranging from 9 to 54. Higher scores indicate higher well-being in each dimension. Internal consistency for these scales was acceptable, ranging from .65 (Autonomy) to .75 (Environmental Mastery).

- *Spirituality.* The Spirituality Assessment Scale (SAS; Howden, 2000) is a 28-item self-report instrument constructed to measure four critical attributes of spirituality (e.g., Purpose and Meaning in Life, Inner Resources, Unifying Interconnectedness, and Transcendence). The SAS employs a 6-point response format ranging from Strongly Disagree to Strongly Agree (with no neutral option). The SAS is scored by summing the responses to all 28 items; each of the four subscale scores may also be obtained by summing the responses of the subscale items. The total scale has a range from 28 to 168. The total instrument was found to have high internal consistency in the ROAH sample (α = .96). The four subscales were found to have acceptably high internal consistency, ranging from α = .82 for Transcendence to α = .91 for Inner Resources.

- *HIV-related stigma.* The HIV Stigma Scale (Berger, 2001) is a 40-item instrument to measure the stigma perceived by people with HIV. Analyses from previous studies of diverse samples of people living with HIV have identified four factors (e.g., Personalized Stigma, Disclosure Concerns, Negative Self-Image, and Concern with Public Attitudes toward People with HIV) and an overall summary score. Scores on the total scale range from 40 to 160, with higher scores indicating greater perceived stigma. Coefficient alphas for the subscales between .83 (Disclosure Concerns) and .95 (Personalized Stigma) and .96 for the total 40-item instrument indicate a high level of internal consistency in the ROAH sample.

- *Disclosure of HIV serostatus.* Disclosure was assessed with an 8-item index used in previous studies of older adults with HIV (Shippy & Karpiak, 2005a, 2005b). Respondents indicate how many people from various groups of individuals (e.g., family, friends, co-workers, sex partners, drug buddies, social/political organizations, healthcare providers, people at place of worship) are aware of their HIV status by marking one of four (i.e.,., none, a few, some or all) levels of disclosure. Participants indicated reasons for non-disclosure on a checklist of common reasons for withholding information about one's HIV status from important others. Responses ranged from "I'm afraid they might kill me" to "They have too many other things to worry about now."

REFERENCES

Cantor, M. H. (1979). Neighbors and friends: An overlooked resource in the informal support system. *Research on Aging, 1,* 434-463.

Cantor, M. H., & Brennan, M. (1993). Family and community support systems of older New Yorkers. *Growing older in New York City in the 1990s: A study of changing lifestyles, quality of life, and quality of care, Vol. V.* New York: New York Center for Policy on Aging, New York Community Trust.

Cantor, M. H., Brennan, M., & Shippy, R. A. (2004). *Caregiving among older lesbian, gay, bisexual, and transgender New Yorkers.* Final report. Washington, DC: National Gay and Lesbian Task Force Policy Institute.

Radloff, L.S. (1977). The CES-D scale: A self report depression scale for research in the general population. *Applied Psychological Measurement, 1,* 385-401.

Russell, D.W. (1996). UCLA Loneliness Scale (Version 3): Reliability, validity and factor structure. *Journal of Personality Assessment, 66*(1), 20-40.

Ryff, C. D., & Essex, M. J. (1992). The interpretation of life experience and well-being: The sample case of relocation. *Psychology and Aging, 7*(4), 507-17.

Shippy, R. A., & Karpiak, S. E. (2005a). The aging HIV/AIDS population: Fragile social networks. *Aging and Mental Health, 9*(3), 246-54.

Shippy, R.A., & Karpiak, S.E. (2005b). Perceptions of support among older adults with HIV. *Research on Aging, 27*(3), 290-306.

Wu, A.W., Rubin, H.R., Mathews, W.C., Ware Jr, J.E., Brysk, L.T., Hardy, W. D., (1991). A health status questionnaire using 30 items from the Medical Outcomes Study. Preliminary validation in persons with early HIV infection. *Medical Care*, 29, 786-798.

INDEX

I

J

85, 86, 87, 89, 90, 92, 93, 94, 96, 100, 101, 102, 106, 107, 110, 111, 114
stigmatization, 62, 106
stigmatized, 60, 73, 91
strain, 31, 49
strains, 30, 40, 47, 93
strategies, 3, 50
streams, 98
strength, 82
stress, 30, 32, 93
stressors, 59
stroke, 20, 107
students, 98
subgroups, 11, 24, 37, 57, 77, 109
subjective, 85
subjective well-being, 85
substance use, viii, ix, xiv, 5, 27, 32, 33, 35, 37, 38, 39, 40, 41, 42, 47, 50, 51, 99, 106, 111, 113
substances, viii, 35, 37, 40, 47, 113
successful aging, 7, 81, 82, 85, 86, 99
suffering, 18, 90
sugar, 20
suicidal ideation, 77, 78
supervision, 15
support services, 65, 100
suppression, 41
Surgeon General, 33
surprise, 59
surveillance, 12, 103
survival, 74
survivors, 97
susceptibility, 33
switching, 18
symptom, 27, 112
symptoms, viii, ix, 15, 17, 24, 27, 28, 30, 32, 33, 40, 48, 49, 59, 77, 79, 84, 93, 96, 112
syndrome, 20
syphilis, 49
systems, ix, 24, 49, 61, 74, 98, 100, 114
systolic blood pressure, 19

T

T cell, viii, 13, 14
T cells, 14
teachers, xiii
telephone, 63, 64, 66, 110, 112
tenure, 105
testimony, viii, 27
testosterone levels, 19
test-retest reliability, 113
therapy, vii, viii, 1, 20, 22, 24, 25, 31, 33, 35, 40, 41, 95, 96

threshold, 28
time frame, 14
tissue, 24, 98
tobacco, 113
tolerance, 20
toxicity, 14
trade, 40
training, 49, 86, 100, 101, 106
training programs, 101
transcendence, x, 87
transcriptase, 17
transformation, 74
transmission, ix, 3, 14, 41, 43, 48, 51, 77
transportation, 90
trauma, 20, 80
treatable, vii, ix, 1, 20, 30, 51
treatment programs, 3, 40
treatment-resistant, 30, 40, 93
triglycerides, 20
tumors, 21

U

UK, 59, 107
underlying mechanisms, 78
uniform, 37
United Nations, 107
United States, 1, 12, 31, 33, 42, 49, 50, 59, 94, 95, 109
universities, 98
upload, 103
urban centers, 3
urinary, 18
urinary tract infection, 18

V

vaccine, 18, 21
vagina, 48
validation, xiv, 25, 115
validity, xiv, 59, 78, 114
values, ix, 28, 75, 82
variable, vii, 13
variables, 7
vascular disease, 19, 20
veterans, 109
violence, 32, 53, 56, 57
viral infection, 49
virus, ix, 3, 14, 17, 19, 20, 21, 24, 30, 31, 33, 40, 49, 50, 51, 77, 84, 93, 98, 101
virus infection, 50
viruses, 40